Return to Mic
of Me
Betty Pe[illegible]

Prevention: The Michigan Experience

The *Prevention in Human Services* series:

- *Evaluation & Prevention in Human Services,* edited by Jared Hermalin and Jonathan A. Morell
- *Helping People to Help Themselves: Self-Help and Prevention,* edited by Leonard D. Borman, Leslie Borck, Robert Hess, and Frank L. Pasquale
- *Early Intervention Programs for Infants,* edited by Howard A. Moss, Robert Hess, and Carolyn Swift
- R_x *Television: Enhancing the Preventive Impact of TV,* edited by Joyce Sprafkin, Carolyn Swift, and Robert Hess
- *Innovations in Prevention,* edited by Robert Hess and Jared Hermalin
- *Strategies for Needs Assessment in Prevention,* edited by Alex Zautra, Kenneth Bachrach, and Robert Hess
- *Aging and Prevention: New Approaches for Preventing Health and Mental Health Problems in Older Adults,* edited by Sharon Simson, Laura B. Wilson, Jared Hermalin, and Robert Hess
- *Studies in Empowerment: Steps Toward Understanding and Action,* edited by Julian Rappaport, Carolyn Swift, and Robert Hess
- *Prevention: The Michigan Experience,* edited by Betty Tableman and Robert Hess
- *Beyond the Individual: Environmental Approaches and Prevention,* edited by Abraham Wandersman and Robert Hess

Prevention: The Michigan Experience

Edited by
Betty Tableman and Robert Hess

The Haworth Press
New York

Prevention: The Michigan Experience has also been published as *Prevention in Human Services,* Volume 3, Number 4, Summer 1985.

The Haworth Press, Inc., 28 East 22 Street, New York, NY 10010

Library of Congress Cataloging in Publication Data
Main entry under title:

Prevention, the Michigan experience.

"Has also been published as Prevention in human services, volume 3, number 4, summer 1985"—T. p. verso.
Includes bibliographies.
1. Community mental health services—Michigan—Addresses, essays, lectures. 2. Mental illness—Prevention—Addresses, essays, lectures. 3. Child mental health services—Michigan—Addresses, essays, lectures. I. Tableman, Betty. II. Hess, Robert, 1948-
RA790.65.M5P74 1985 362.2'0425 85-8071
ISBN 0-86656-458-6

Prevention: The Michigan Experience

Prevention in Human Services
Volume 3, Number 4

CONTENTS

ACKNOWLEDGMENT

With special appreciation to C. Patrick Babcock, Director of the Michigan Department of Mental Health, for his strong support of prevention efforts in the state.

Introduction

Robert E. Hess

Before coming to Michigan, I often heard about the solid work being done in the field of prevention by Betty Tableman and the Michigan Department of Mental Health. As a result, one of the first calls I made after arriving in the state several years ago was to Betty. This was the beginning of a series of contacts which led to my becoming a member of the Advisory Committee on Prevention and Community/Caregiver Services and to the development of an intimate knowledge of Michigan's prevention efforts.

I have been impressed by what I have seen in Michigan and believe readers can gain much from an in-depth look at what has been done. I should note that because this volume is devoted to Michigan it should not be assumed that other states do not have excellent models; many of them do. The purpose of this volume is to use Michigan to illustrate what a state can do to further prevention and to highlight some areas that are unique to the Michigan model. Information of a practical nature is also provided which might be of use to those working in field settings.

There are many aspects of the Michigan model which I find noteworthy but a few, in particular, stand out in my mind. First, I am impressed with the ecological soundness of the pilot demonstration concept. Programs, such as interpersonal cognitive problem solving, which have been well-researched and found to be effective elsewhere are not assumed to be effective in Michigan because of possible differences in settings. Rather than being adopted without close study, as so often happens, such programs are piloted and then replicated with research being conducted to determine whether or not they are effective within the context of Michigan's mental health system.

That these pilots and replications even have a research component, let alone a well-designed one, is impressive when one considers that the bulk of these studies are conducted in community mental health centers by staff with little research experience.

Having spent over a decade in community mental health centers, I can attest to the fact that conducting research is far from the norm in these settings because of constraints in resources. Given this, I am prone to overlook problems that occurred during the course of some of these studies and have nothing but praise for those who had the courage to undertake them.

Also worthy of note is the existence of a policy within the Department of Mental Health to allow programs to receive ongoing continuation funding once they have been found to be successful. This policy has the effect of institutionalizing prevention within community mental health services while freeing up funds for the development of new projects. Thus, prevention is mainstreamed rather than remaining on the very vulnerable fringes.

The use of advisory groups in the Michigan model is another noteworthy feature. Advisory groups increased the probability that prevention programs will be responsive to constituents while making them less vulnerable to the very real possibility of funding cuts. The membership of these groups consists primarily of professionals but it is my hope that they will add consumers and evolve to the point where they provide an avenue for consumer empowerment. Given the trend toward consumerism in Michigan, this hope is not without foundation.

The existence of a state effort on behalf of prevention has done much to further the development of prevention services on a local level in Michigan. Michigan is not alone in having such an effort; as Betty Tableman states in her overview, there are a number of states with similar efforts. However, there are a number of states that do not have such efforts. It is hoped that this volume will serve as an impetus for readers to work with their states so that, in time, they will develop models to assist local communities in furthering prevention.

Overview of Michigan Prevention Programming

Betty Tableman
Michigan Department of Mental Health

ABSTRACT. The Michigan Department of Mental Health's prevention programming has centered around the development of community service models through pilot demonstration projects. A systems approach has resulted in the formulation of departmental guidelines and policies. Pilot demonstration projects have been directed primarily at enhancing coping skills of high risk populations. Collaborative interagency efforts have provided an additional dimension to Michigan prevention programming.

Michigan is one of a growing number of states which have set aside a small amount of resources for prevention programming. Prevention activity, directed toward at-risk populations and health promotion, has developed idiosyncratically in state departments of mental health, reflecting not only the state of the art but political and organizational imperatives unique to the particular situation.

Some states have assigned funds to local prevention services without specific state level prevention staff. Other states have assigned state level staff to prevention programming but have not yet made funds available for services. A few states have assigned both funds and staff. Along another dimension, a few states limit their programming to a single component (e.g., social support in California, infants in Maine, children in disordered families in New York). Most states, however, are eclectic in their range of concerns (Tableman, in press).

Michigan has had prevention programming since 1976, with both state level staff and funding. This issue of *Prevention in Human Services* provides an opportunity to review the Michigan experience.

Reprints are available from Betty Tableman, Michigan Department of Mental Health, Lewis Cass Building, Lansing, MI 48926.

This overview will describe the background, including administrative parameters and basic concepts, and areas of development for the Michigan program, so as to provide a context for the articles which follow.

BACKGROUND

The Michigan Department of Mental Health's prevention programming derives from the Mental Health Code's recognition of prevention as a community mental health activity. In 1975, the director of the Department acceded to the concerns of the Mental Health Association in Michigan that the provisions of the new code be implemented; he requested a position paper on the assumption that public health-type preventive interventions were being overlooked. A six month exploration found no such initiatives but instead a few promising areas of generative research. On the strength of recommendations which charted the course programmatically and administratively (Tableman, 1975), the director assigned staff resources and obtained an appropriation for pilot demonstration projects. Despite four changes in administrations and economic cutbacks, the program has been sustained, with an elaboration over time in both programmatic concerns and administrative parameters. A systems approach has been taken to the development of service models and to the installation of prevention as a programmatic component.

ADMINISTRATIVE PARAMETERS

Administratively, there have been three constant elements in the Michigan Department of Mental Health's prevention programming: as advisory committee, a program unit, and a legislative appropriation for project development. The advisory committee's essential role is described in the article by Floyd Smith, its current chairperson, and Robert Hess. The prevention function has been variously placed within the department over the years, reporting initially to the deputy director of the department. Currently the prevention function is located within the Research and Evaluation Division, Bureau of Clinical and Medical Services. Despite organizational shifts, basic staffing and direction have remained stable. The staff, ranging from one to three persons, currently stands at two full-time equivalent, plus secretarial support.

The legislative appropriation, initiated in 1976 with $400,000, currently provides around $800,000 for prevention projects. In addition, funds have been provided since 1982 to permit transfer of projects to continuation funding.

Developmental Cycle

Projects are defined as pilot demonstrations; this initially permitted development of community service models without requiring a departmental commitment to prevention. Pilot demonstration projects are evaluated with an experimental and control group. When the service model is considered viable, it is the intent to replicate it in another setting, again with an evaluation component. Beyond this stage, the model is installed in other community mental health boards as a dissemination project, without an evaluation component but with an ongoing feedback measure. Dissemination projects are retained on project funding for one year to assure that they are running satisfactorily and then transferred to regular community mental health funding.

Prevention service models are documented in a replication manual. The documentation forces clarification of the model's characteristics and components, and the availability of the manual facilitates translation into other settings.

Departmental Guidelines

As external support for prevention programming has become evident, and as the projects have been validated through evaluation results and community response, a gradually evolving commitment has been expressed through explicit formulations of departmental policy. Administrative manual guidelines, providing sanction and definition, have been adopted for prevention services as a community mental health component and for services provided to community agencies and infant mental health services as expressions of that component. An administrative manual guideline on continuation and transfer of projects provides the framework for initial development and ongoing departmental support of prevention services. If the community mental health board expresses its intent to continue the prevention projects as an ongoing service, the department increases the support base for the board to include the prevention service. The board is obligated to continue the prevention service for three years and cannot transfer the funds provided. Funds are assigned in the community mental health appropriation to underwrite this transfer.

Prevention services are included in departmental rules and regulations as a mandated community service. The department initially granted community mental health boards a general waiver of the mandate. In 1983 that policy was rescinded, and community mental health boards without prevention services are now required to request a waiver annually. Boards seeking full management status (i.e., assuming full responsibility for all mental health services to their residents in exchange for increased fiscal flexibility) are expected to provide prevention services. The route for the development of prevention services continues to be through projects under the line item appropriation with subsequent transfer to regular community mental health funding.

Administrative Concepts

The Michigan program developed in response to a legislative authorization for community-based prevention services, and its basic objective has been to implement that legislative authorization. Early decisions in support of that objective have shaped the Michigan program.

The decisions to undertake projects through community mental health and to require a local match were consistent with customary departmental operations and avoided making projects fiscally as well as programmatically special.

The decision to fund many small projects spread the risk, built a constituency, and allowed a wider range of experimentation. Whenever possible, projects have been paired, again spreading the risk and providing insight through comparison.

The decision to define projects as pilot demonstrations and to evaluate them required a commitment to allocate funds for data collection, processing, and analysis. The department has taken responsibility for the evaluation design and for data analysis, except in those few instances where the community mental health board had an evaluator on staff. Implementation and data collection have been the responsibility of the project staff. Evaluations thus have been undertaken in the context of community-based field research with all of its limitations and uncertainties (Cowen, 1978). Department staff have become sensitive to the need for oversight and technical assistance in assuring random assignment, minimizing attrition, and managing data.

An early pragmatic decision was to focus on proximal outcomes. The problems of small samples and attrition over time, cost considerations, and the short-term decision lines of state agencies, have all operated against follow-up studies.

The evaluation report was initially conceptualized as a decision point, requiring clear evidence of impact for continuation of efforts. However, experience with the limitations of evaluation methodology has somewhat shifted the emphasis. Evaluation is now conceptualized as a means of reviewing and reorienting efforts, of adding to the store of information about the intervention and the population. Evaluations thus routinely include an assessment of process and anecdotal evidence of impact, as well as outcome measures.

AREAS OF PROGRAMMING

Pilot demonstration projects have evolved from both local initiative and from areas of interest defined by the department. Risk factor research has been used to define populations and intervention issues; clinical and methodological research and clinical experience have shaped intervention approaches.

Infant Mental Health Services

The department's support for infant mental health services dates from 1973 and 1974 when Fraiberg's Infant Development Project, University of Michigan, was funded for extension training in the concepts and practice of infant mental health (Shapiro, Adelson, & Tableman, 1982). The provision of training for twelve community clinicians led to immediate service development in a few mental health centers. The availability of funding for prevention projects facilitated the translation of this training into service development.

Through 1984, there have been infant mental health and adolescent parent projects in 14 areas, 11 of which have become or are becoming viable ongoing services. In addition, there have been two major by-products: the hospital-based screener, described in the article by Tableman and Katzenmeyer, and the Objectives/Problems Checklist, an outline that provides a way of capturing the problem profile and progress made in infant cases. An unforeseen consequence of the Department's infant programming, the Michigan Association for Infant Mental Health, is described in the article by Fitzgerald.

Parent Training

A parent training model for low-income families with preschool children is described in the article by Mischley, Stacy, Mischley, and Dush. Another parent training project, using a social learning approach, is directed at prevention of conduct disorders in young children of alcoholic parents; the evaluation will assess change in both parents and children.

Interpersonal Cognitive Problem-Solving Training

The article by Feis and Simons describes an evaluation of the Shure model replicated in a Headstart program in rural Newaygo county. In addition, an ICPS manual has been developed for use with children of disordered adults.

Stress Management Training for Low-Income Women

The stress management training model, a major contribution of the Michigan program, is described in the article by Tableman, Feis, Howard, and Marciniak.

Community Model

The article by Tableman, Marciniak, and Bissell describes the components of a community model of prevention services which derives from experiences in Ionia and Newaygo counties.

Other Projects

Children of disordered adults. In view of risk studies indicating the vulnerability of children attached to mentally ill parents, services for children of disordered adults were an early area of development. Infant mental health services include mentally ill parents as a subset of families served, and infant projects have been encouraged to develop linkages with adult mental health services. The children of disordered adults projects, however, have concentrated on elementary-age and adolescent children attached to adult clients, attempting to mediate the impact of parental disorder on the child. An outreach model is used, with elements of crisis intervention, interpretation to the child and to the parents, problem-solving training, resource linkage, advocacy with the schools and training of parents in child management skills. One successful project and two abortive attempts suggest that success in undertaking this type of programming depends on the ability of project staff to function in a broad outreach model and on the viability of the referral and collaborative linkages between adult services and the children's project.

Children of divorce. Two current projects are evaluating different approaches to the children of divorce. One recruits families through the circuit court, attempting to reach parents and children during the early stages of the divorce process. Three approaches are being evaluated: a single educational session for parents, eight session psycho-educational group for parents and for children, and family mediation. The second project views adaptation to divorce as an ongoing process and enrolls children at various stages in the divorce experience for a school-based group intervention.

Unemployment. An early project replicated Azrin's Job Finding Club (Azrin, Flores, & Kaplan, 1975). Although the record on job placement corroborated Azrin's findings, a smoothly functioning referral process was not implemented, and the project was dropped. Subsequently, the 1980 economic recession led to a further exploration of the impact of joblessness. A book of readings was assembled to provide basic information to community mental health agencies. A manual was developed for mental health centers confronted with plant closings and mass layoffs as a result of the interest of a metropolitan area mental health center director.

Resource Development

Although the legislative appropriation has been used primarily to fund service development at the community level, it has also made possible the development of resource materials and instruments and the underwriting of infant mental health training. All of these activities are designed to contribute toward local service development.

Self-help. Although mutual support has been encouraged in some projects, the department's programming has only recently begun a serious exploration of the self-help dimension of prevention programming. A manual directed at community mental health agencies in Michigan has been commissioned, and the feasibility of establishing a statewide clearinghouse is being assessed.

Prevention of secondary depression. A current project is developing informational materials for physicians and other health care professionals concerning the impact of certain drugs and medications on individuals with a past or familial history of depression.

Community/caregiver services. A continuing minor theme has been the conceptualization of community/caregiver services. In response to interest and concern expressed by advisory committee members, the consultation/education component relating to both prevention and client populations has been explored, resulting in the development of departmental guidelines for community/caregiver services. Special projects have piloted and operationalized the departmental guidelines as well as an appropriate management information system.

Interagency Collaboration

While Michigan's prevention programming has focused on the development of community service models, collaborative efforts have added an important dimension. Prevention staff has played a policy role in various interagency planning and service arrangements. These have included the Interdisciplinary Prevention Council which puts on an annual conference, various interagency committees to develop services for pregnant adolescents and adolescent parents, the steering committee for the Michigan Model for Comprehensive School Health Education, and the executive committee of the Michigan Preventive Intervention Research Center. (The Michigan Preventive Intervention Research Center, a federally funded research effort directed at unemployment issues, is described in the article by Price.) Participation in these efforts has been productive for broader prevention interests and illuminating as case studies of service development within the context of collaborative arrangements.

THE FUTURE

Over eight years, Michigan's prevention programming has moved from exploratory pilot projects to the formulation of service models, from prevention as a special project initiative to prevention as an integral part of community mental health programming. This has occurred within the national context of a rapidly developing critical mass of research and greater visibility and emphasis on prevention at the federal level. In Michigan the context has involved individual and organizational support outside the department and a willingness to move forward on the part of key decisionmakers within the department.

What of the future? Clearly the Michigan program is entering a phase during which the emphasis must shift from pilot demonstration and model development to replication and dissemination. The major share of available funding must be directed toward installing prevention programming in those community mental health boards currently under waiver before embarking on a second round for those motivated boards who participated in the initial pilot projects. Within the department we might expect prevention programming directed at high-risk infants and children of disordered adults to be implemented as part of the emerging continuum of children's services.

Programmatically, we expect to continue the effort to understand the strengths and weaknesses of each of our program models. We expect more attention to be directed at formulating a community continuum and at assessing the trade-offs between interventions at early and subsequent ages.

Finally, the changing milieu for prevention programming in Michigan will also result in greater emphasis at the state level on interdepartmental efforts and collaborative programming. The organization, for example, of trust funds for the prevention of child abuse and neglect and for health-promotion/risk-reduction activities provides opportunities for translating and disseminating program models and concepts.

REFERENCES

Azrin, N., Flores, T., & Kaplan, S.J. (1975). Job finding club: A group-assisted program for obtaining employment. *Behavior Research and Therapy, 13,* 17-27.

Cowen, E.L. (1978). Some problems in community program evaluation research. *Journal of Consulting and Clinical Psychology, 46,* 792-805.

Shapiro, V., Adelson, E., & Tableman, B. (1982). The introduction of infant mental health services in Michigan. *Infant Mental Health Journal, 3,* 69-139.

Tableman, B. (1975). *Recommendations on the development of a prevention system.* Lansing: Michigan Department of Mental Health.

Tableman, B. (in press). The politics of the possible. In M. Kessler & S. Goldston (Eds.), *Proceedings of the Tenth Annual Vermont Conference on Prevention of Psychopathology.* Hanover: University of New Hampshire Press.

The Role of the Prevention Advisory Committee in Michigan

Floyd Smith
AuSable Valley Community Mental Health

Robert Hess
Riverwood Community Mental Health Center

ABSTRACT. The role of a prevention advisory committee in maintaining Michigan's prevention effort is examined. Accomplishments in the areas of program development, communication, policy formulation, and advocacy are described and structural aspects contributing to the success of the committee are discussed.

Prevention services are vulnerable services. Despite data showing the effectiveness of a range of prevention services, they are criticized by traditionalists (Lamb & Zussman, 1979). In mental health agencies, prevention services are vulnerable because administrators are under pressure to assign limited resources to services for those with problems as opposed to those at risk of problems. As a result, prevention services are under financed and generally the first services to be eliminated in the event of fiscal difficulties.

Because they are vulnerable, prevention services require a vigilant and vocal constituency. Within a state system, such as the Michigan Department of Mental Health, attention tends to gravitate to major issues and ongoing crises. An outside constituency is essential to support departmental efforts and to work to further prevention as a field.

Floyd Smith is the current chair of the Michigan Advisory Committee on Prevention and Community/Caregiver Services. Robert Hess is a member of the committee. Reprints may be obtained from the first author at AuSable Valley Community Mental Health, 1199 West Harris Avenue, P.O. Box 310, Tawas City, MI 48763.

In Michigan, a prevention advisory committee has been a significant component of this constituency. The committee has been in existence since the beginning of the state's prevention effort and has served as an advocate for prevention programs, a communications link for those in the field, and a shaper of policy in the area of prevention. It has played a crucial role in the continuity and stability of prevention programs in Michigan.

HISTORY

The roots of the prevention advisory committee can be traced to an ad hoc group constituted in late 1974 by the director of the Department of Mental Health to develop recommendations for departmental efforts in the area of prevention. The ad hoc committee presented 19 recommendations in June of 1975 (Tableman, 1975) including a recommendation that a permanent advisory committee be established.

The director of the Department accepted the recommendations of the ad hoc committee, initiated a prevention program, and established a permanent advisory committee. The committee was given the following charge:

> The role of the Committee is to review the procedures and operational policies of the Prevention System, to advise on the direction of development, to provide to the Prevention System an assessment of the way in which its activities affect community operations, and to interpret to commumty agencies the direction and actions of the Prevention System. In essence the Committee's function is to assure that the Prevention System is accountable and responsive to the field constituency while remaining responsible to the Director of the Department. (Michigan Department of Mental Health, 1976, p.1)

The prevention advisory committee held its first meeting on April 7, 1976 and has continued to meet every other month on a regular basis. In its 9 years of existence, it has had strong support from and extensive interaction with the unit in the Department of Mental Health responsible for prevention programming. Through this partnership it has significantly contributed to the advancement of prevention services in Michigan.

ACCOMPLISHMENTS

Development and Dissemination

The prevention advisory committee has supported and contributed to the development of pilot demonstration projects. Of particular importance has been the emphasis the committee has placed on evaluation. Committee members with expertise in research methodology have encouraged the development of the strongest possible evaluation component.

When evaluation results have been positive, the committee has provided strong support for development of the replication manual and program dissemination. The committee has had a special interest in suggesting methods for dissemination at times when fiscal or other barriers have curtailed efforts in this area.

Communication

The advisory committee has served as a forum for the discussion and assessment of new ideas in prevention. One of the major problems in the development of prevention as a field has been a lack of communication between practitioners and others in the mental health field. Cognizant of this problem, the committee has developed several methods to ensure communication within the department and among individuals interested in prevention.

The committee reminds the department of its presence by circulating minutes of its meetings to departmental executive staff. This communication also serves to keep these staff members aware of the current status of the department's prevention effort.

Committee meetings link practitioners, researchers, and state agency staff together so that they not only bring their unique perceptions to bear on issues but also share information and learn from one another. This has raised the level of awareness of members and has served to disseminate prevention information. Moreover, the relationships established in the advisory committee have facilitated the development of other interactions.

Finally, the committee has been one of the sponsors of an annual interdisciplinary prevention conference which provides an opportunity for professionals from a wide variety of fields to share information and to learn about the latest developments in the field of prevention. Most presentations at this conference are given by practitioners in the state, thus making it easier for those in attendance to receive consultation on an ongoing basis if they decide to implement one of the featured programs.

Departmental Policy

The key area of involvement for the prevention advisory committee has been in the developmemt of departmental policy. The committee's work has affected the development of guidelines, the removal of a service waiver, and the establishment of funding processes. All have been critical steps toward institutionalizing prevention within the range of mental health services in Michigan.

The committee has been deeply involved in the development of guidelines under which state-funded prevention and community/caregiver services are operated. The Department of Mental Health, like most state departments, often issues guidelines which fail to take into account the realities of field settings. The advisory committee, because of the inclusion of professionals from applied settings in its membership, has been able to assist in the development of realistic prevention guidelines. Equally important, the committee has developed strategies for the presentation of the guidelines to the field which has resulted in a broad base of support for adoption and implementation.

Although prevention services are required of community mental health centers by Michigan statute, funding constraints and the initiation of the pilot demonstration process resulted in the issuance of a blanket waiver by the Department of Mental Health. The committee believed that this blanket waiver reduced the status of prevention services. When evaluated community models became available, the committee took the initiative and was instrumental in having the blanket waiver rescinded. The net effect has been to increase substantially the perceived importance of prevention, not only in community mental health centers but also in the department itself.

Another major accomplishment of the committee was the development of a mechanism for continued funding of prevention services after the pilot phase. The prevention unit of the department operates as a project granting unit under a special legislative appropriation. Successful prevention programs thus were not ensured of funding beyond the period of their development grant. The committee met with the director of the department to explore how continuation funding might be provided. The result was the development of departmental guidelines through which the department agreed to transfer to continuation funding any prevention project which was found to be effective. The assurance of continuation funding has resulted in development of a strong prevention presence in a number of the community mental health centers. Prevention projects have, in essence, become institutionalized as community mental health services.

A critical element of this agreement with the department was that as projects were transferred, the budget of the prevention unit would be sustained. Without this element, the unit would have quickly gone out of business, a victim of its own success. With this agreement, the unit is able to develop new pilot and replication programs and spin them off to continuation funding, with the expectation of being able to repeat the process for other new programs.

Advocacy

Advocacy has been a key role of the committee in recent years. Prevention programs have been especially vulnerable to budget cuts as Michigan has experienced its worst financial period since the depression. Prevention funding was cut but, because of continuing advocacy on the part of the advisory committee and community groups, no projects were actually lost. This record is noteworthy as other special programming developed by the department was not sustained.

Earlier, the committee played an equally important role in advocating for the maintenance of infant mental health projects, when they were in jeopardy because of ambiguous evaluation results. When departmental research staff wanted to eliminate them, the advisory committee established a specially qualified subcommittee to review the projects and the evaluation design. The subcommittee recommended changes and the projects were continued with a more appropriate evaluation. The value of these projects has been demonstrated, and they are now considered among the most successful of Michigan's prevention efforts.

DISCUSSION

The prevention advisory committee has met with marked success in its roles of developer, advocate, and communicator. It has been integral to the development and maintenance of prevention efforts in

Michigan. Its presence has blunted the benign neglect of some directors of the department and enhanced the supportive activities of other directors. Because of the importance of the committee to the Michigan program, it is worthwhile to discuss some of the elements that have made it successful.

One of the important elements in the continuing success of the committee has been the quality of membership. Consistently, six to eight of the strongest and most respected community mental health directors in the state have been members. The committee has also included well respected representatives from other state departments, voluntary organizations, and the major universities in the state. The advisory committee has drawn on persons with prior experience and expertise in prevention services; it has also provided a means of expanding the number of persons with a knowledge of and investment in prevention.

This particular spread of membership has provided credibility with community mental health centers and the Department of Mental Health. It has also provided access to the legislature at times when such access was vital to a strong prevention presence within the state. A member of the original advisory committee observed that in seeking committee members, the head of the prevention unit "had the guts to go for people with clout."

Additional clout stems from the fact that appointments to the committee are made by the director of the Department of Mental Health. This provides a greater sense of credibility and assurance of access to the director.

Another element which has given strength to the committee has been strong continuity among key members. The committee, during its 9 years, has had only two chairs. There are still several members who were among the original appointments to the ad hoc committee. In some circumstances, such lack of turnover leads to paresis. In the case of the advisory committee, it has provided some sense of history and continuity within the committee and it has been a strength rather than a weakness.

A final element that has contributed to the success of the committee has been the fact that it has had a close, productive relationship with the department's prevention unit. There has been a true partnership with all parties working to further prevention in the state of Michigan. The committee has been important to the department in bringing resources to the development of prevention programming. In turn, the department has been important to the committee members by providing a mechanism for professionals with a deep commitment to prevention to see their ideas and efforts come to fruition.

REFERENCES

Lamb, H.R., & Zusman, J. (1979). Primary prevention in perspective. *American Journal of Psychiatry, 136,* 12-17.

Michigan Department of Mental Health (1976, April). *Minutes of prevention system advisory committee.* Author: Lansing, MI.

Tableman, B. (1975). *Development of a prevention system* (Report to Donald C. Smith, M.D., Acting Director). Lansing: Michigan Department of Mental Health.

Infant Mental Health Services: A Newborn Screener

Betty Tableman
Michigan Department of Mental Health

Muriel Katzenmeyer
Kalamazoo County Mental Health Services Board

ABSTRACT. In order to identify newborns at psychosocial risk so that intervention could be provided proactively, a screener was developed for use by nurses in the hospital. The situational and interactional content of the screener are described. The screener was validated against 1 month and 1 year scores on measures assessing the environment and parent-infant interaction. Correlations with 1 year data suggest predictive validity.

The Michigan Department of Mental Health's infant programming is derived from Fraiberg's (1980) home visit model, characterized as "psychotherapy in the kitchen." Initially these infant mental health services operated on a traditional referral basis: professionals referred families in distress where the impact of aberrant parenting on infants and toddlers was already evident. As the infant specialists worked with these families, they found that they could educate professionals to become more sensitive to mother-infant interaction and early signs of dyssynchrony and stress. It seemed appropriate to seek a systematic way of identifying infants in situations that placed them at risk so that referrals could be made, not after the fact, but proactively during the early months of life.

The development of a screening instrument rests on an assump-

---

The BIA was developed at the Early Intervention Program, Borgess Pediatric Center, P.C., and piloted at Borgess Hospital, Kalamazoo. Those responsible for its development include: Don Johnson, Louise Woodhams, Jan Barnes, Jan Goertz, Jerry Ferguson, and Betty Tableman. Muriel Katzenmeyer was responsible for the evaluation. Data were collected by Vicki Johnson, Susan Ordway, and Barbara Gilbert

Reprints are available from Betty Tableman, Michigan Department of Mental Health, Lewis Cass Building, Lansing, MI, 48926.

tion of continuity, i.e., that in the absence of positive life changes or effective intervention the interactional patterns perceived at birth are congruent with those evident at 1 year and will continue. Although there has been considerable discontinuity over time in measures of the infant related to outcome, Sroufe has found stability in stage-appropriate indices of parent-infant attachment and parenting behavior (Sroufe, 1979).

Department of Mental Health support for the development of a newborn screener was energized by a medical care practice in Kalamazoo County. Their request to the Kalamazoo County Mental Health Services Board for assistance in identifying and intervening with infants in nurturing situations indicative of psycho-social risk resulted in the Early Intervention Program piloting a proactive, systematic approach to infant mental health. The project had two components: screening mother-infant dyads for indices of risk and intervening with those identified as presumed high risk.

The screening instrument, the Borgess Interaction Assessment (BIA), was developed after a review of several similar efforts at identification of high-risk infants. The department's interest in developing community service models required an instrument that could be installed in the average hospital. This argued for a simply administered instrument which could systematize the hospital nurses' observations and referral judgments. In addition, the instrument had to discriminate reliably between high-risk and low-risk dyads, and the judgments made had to be consistent with later information justifying the determination made.

An attitudinal measure to assess propensity for abuse (Helfer & Schneider, 1975) was reviewed and discarded as too intrusive to be acceptable as a routine part of hospital operations. Broussard's (1979) Neonatal Perception Inventory (NPI) was carefully considered. The Neonatal Perception Inventory taps the mother's perception of her baby versus the average baby, at 1 day and 1 month, with respect to six items: crying, spitting, feeding, elimination, sleeping, and predictability. The score is obtained by determining the discrepancy between the mother's two ratings, suggesting a dissonance if she perceives her infant as less than average. The NPI was validated by having a psychiatrist blind to the ratings assess the children at 4 1/2 years and 10-11 years. This research indicated early negative perceptions by a mother were predictive of later assessment of mental disorder. While the simplicity of the NPI was attractive, its predictability depended upon 1 month ratings. The first rating alone was not predictive, and the instability between a mother's perception recorded during her hospital stay and that obtained at 1 month made the NPI inappropriate as a hospital-based screening mechanism.

We turned then to the experience of Gray, Cutler, Dean, and Kempe (1977), observing the reaction of mothers to their infants in the delivery room. They found that post-delivery observation could identify 76% of the infants who would experience abnormal parenting practices during the first 2 years of life as evidenced by abuse, neglect, injury related to lack of care, failure to thrive, and relinquishment of the infant. However, this post-delivery screening process would not work for Caesarean mothers who constitute as much as 25% of deliveries in Michigan hospitals. For this reason, and because of the interest of the nursery supervisor in Kalamazoo, a parallel observation of interaction during the hospital stay was designed. Some factors cited in the literature as indicative of risk were also included.

DESCRIPTION OF THE BIA

The screener which was developed in the Kalamazoo project thus included both observational factors of affect and responsiveness in parental behavior, and various situational factors which might adversely affect bonding or nurturing behavior. The BIA had three parts: (a) the situational part covering 16 items; (b) the post-delivery part based on observation of the mother's response to the infant, covering 7 items; and (c) the postpartum part, based on observation of the mother's interaction with the infant during the hospital stay, covering 12 items. Information for the situational items was obtained from the medical record and through conversations with the mother. Observation of the mother's interaction was incorporated into the normal routine in the hospital setting. The BIA form was not filled out or scored in front of the mother; it was treated as any other part of observational charting. The BIA was scored on the second day; names of mother-infant dyads receiving high scores were telephoned to the early intervention program so that a contact could be made before the mother left the hospital.

The situational part included some characteristics of the infant which suggest increased vulnerability: low birth weight, low Apgar score, and irritability. It also included the past and present experiences of the mother which may impair bonding: whether she had lost a previous infant, whether her pregnancy was medically high-risk, and whether the infant's or the mother's condition resulted in separation after birth.

Some items were indicative of stressors that can impair nurturance: whether the mother was a single parent, whether the family was unemployed, and whether there were closely spaced siblings. Extra weight was given to the young age of the mother and to a parental history of mental illness, retardation, substance abuse, or child abuse, when this information was known. There were three items on the mother's support system. Other items tapped into attitudes and affect: was the baby wanted, was the mother satisfied with the sex of the baby, had preparations been made, and were there any problems over naming of the baby?

The second and third parts of the screener provided for a systematic observation by nurses of the mother's interaction with the infant. The intrapartum observation was undertaken by a delivery room nurse and captured how the mother reacted to the infant immediately after delivery and during the hospital stay. When the introductory observations could not be made, the items were omitted. The postpartum observation was completed within 48 hours after a vaginal birth by a maternity unit nurse who made her assessment only after she had several opportunities in the course of caregiving to observe the mother's behavior; each contact contributed to the amount and stability of information. In the case of a Caesarean section, assessment was not initiated until the effects of the anaesthesia had worn off.

Items were scored 0 to 2, with 0 being the most favorable condition. A maximum score, without the special weighted items, would be 70. An initial cut-off score of 14 was revised downward to 10 after the pediatric nurse practitioner systematically reviewed medical practice records for families with a score of 10 to 13. With the exceptions noted, the determination of presumed risk was based on a cumulative score: at a cutoff score of 10, five or more situational or observational factors had to be present to suggest risk.

For dyads where post-delivery observation was not possible, the assessment was based on 28 out of 35 items, a reduction of 20%. The cutoff score was therefore lowered by 20%, or 2 points, to 8. To simplify processing for the nurses, 2 points were added. Because two cutoff scores introduced an element of complexity for the nurses, the 2 points were added for dyads lacking post-delivery scores so that the cutoff score remained consistently at 10.

METHOD

Participants

The BIA was installed in Borgess Hospital and Bronson Methodist Hospital, Kalamazoo for all mother-infant dyads served by a group of pediatricians involved concurrently in a hospital-based pediatric clinic and private practice. During a 17 month period, 1062 mother-infant dyads served by these pediatricians were screened, representing about 80% of the births at one hospital and 10% at the other. This represented the entire practice of these pediatricians.

Procedure

Validation of the BIA had three aspects: an assessment of interrater reliability, an analysis of the internal consistency and reliability of the BIA in discriminating between presumed high-risk and presumed low-risk dyads, and determination of predictive validity.

Interrater Reliability

Interrater reliability among the nurses for the observational items was determined after systematic training by having the nurses score videotapes prepared by project staff. Twenty-five labor/delivery nurses and 67 postpartum care nurses participated, almost all of the staff in these areas. The percentage of agreement in rating was calculated by dividing the number of agreements by the total number of items, times the number of participants.

Internal Consistency

Internal consistency of the BIA was established by randomly selecting a representative sample of 200 from the total population of 1062 mother-infant dyads screened and calculating two measures: coefficient alpha for each part score and the total score (Lord & Novick, 1968); and an indicator of predictive association, lambda, for individual items (Hayes, 1973). Coefficient alpha provided an indication of the extent to which the items were measuring the same factor, i.e., risk. The index of predictive association represented the proportional reduction in the probability of error in prediction when item scores were used; thus it provided information on the utility of specific items in the classification of presumed high risk or presumed low risk.

Predictive Validity

Validation of the BIA as a newborn screener rested on the extent to which it selected, at birth, families who in the short-run were exhibiting interactional and nurturing patterns indicative of risk. Thus, predictiveness was determined by testing the hypothesis that groups identified by scores on the BIA at birth would also differ at 1 month and again at 1 year on subsequent measures of parent-infant interaction and characteristics of the environment predictive of competent development. Validation based on longer range outcome data was not attempted within the time and resource constraints of the state program.

Measures. Scores for presumed high-risk and presumed low-risk dyads were compared on three instruments—HOME, NCAF, and NCAT—which measured parent-infant interaction and characteristics of the environment predictive of developmental competence.

The HOME (Home Observation for Measurement of the Environment) had 45 items located on six scales: emotional and verbal responsivity of the mother, avoidance of restriction, organization of the environment, provision of appropriate play material, maternal involvement with the child, and opportunities for variety in daily stimulation. Information for the ratings was obtained by interview and observation. The test was standardized on infants from "normal" and "high-risk" families. Research on the HOME inventory has resulted in internal consistency coefficients ranging from .44 to .89 for the subscales (Caldwell & Bradley, 1978).

The HOME was selected because it contained both interactional and stimulation components: it had been found to be predictive of cognitive development (Bradley & Caldwell, 1978) and of behavioral problems at age 4 (Eyres, Barnard, & Gray, 1980).

Twelve items on the HOME were age-inappropriate. Rather than coding them 0 which would have depressed scores at 1 month, those items were deleted from the interview at 1 month. For comparability, scores were converted to the percentage of items administered at each time that were rated "yes" (positive). This procedure tended to increase the spread between 1 month and 1 year scores in comparison with the other meaures.

The Nursing Child Assessment Feeding Scale (NCAF, 76 items)

and the Nursing Child Assessment Teaching Scale (NCAT, 73 items) were observational instruments which assessed the positive reciprocal relationship between parent and infant during feeding (NCAF) or when the mother taught the infant an age-appropriate game (NCAT). Each scale had two parts: the parent score with four dimensions of maternal behavior (i.e., sensitivity to cues, response to distress, social-emotional growth fostering, and cognitive growth fostering) and the child score with two dimensions of infant behavior (i.e., clarity of cues and responsiveness to parent). The Feeding scale tapped a familiar and often repeated transaction. The Teaching scale was a more novel situation which placed some stress on the mother-infant dyad, thus providing a measure of the adaptive interaction of the dyad.

Internal consistency (Cronbach's alpha) was .83 for both Parent scales, .73 for Child Feeding scales, and .60 for Child Teaching scales. Predictive validity for Bayley Mental Development at 24 months, expressive and receptive language scores at 36 months, Binet IQ at 48 months, and problem behavior at 36 months, based on a small sample, ranged from .30 to .50 for multiple regression equations for the feeding scales and .30 for the teaching scales (Barnard & Bee, 1982).

The NCAF and NCAT were selected because they focused on the repertoire of parent-infant interactional behaviors and could be implemented with good reliability in field settings. While other measures may be richer in assessing parent-infant interaction and attachment behavior (cf., Ainsworth, Blehar, Waters, & Wall, 1978; Greenspan & Lieberman, 1980; Woods, 1975), they require a laboratory situation or a videotaping and rating process beyond Michigan field capabilities.

Procedure. Pairs of presumed high-risk infants (BIA score of 10 or more) were assigned randomly to experimental and control groups for evaluation of the intervention. The next available presumed low-risk infant was selected for comparison in the validity and reliability assessment. Fifty-six families were assigned to each unserved condition; after attrition, data were available for both testing times for 38 presumed high-risk dyads and 39 presumed low-risk dyads. Data were collected in the home on the HOME and NCAF when the infant was 1 month and on all three measures at 1 year of age. The Teaching scale was omitted at 1 month because of the limited capacity of the infant. Data collectors participated in the University of Washington-sponsored Nursing Child Assessment

Scales Training, with reliability established by paired observations; interrater agreement exceeded the 85% recommended. Collectors were blind to the dyad's risk status. Families were paid a nominal sum for data collection.

RESULTS

Distribution of Scores

With a cutoff score of 10, 19.5% of the mother-infant dyads were identified as presumed high risk. Almost 4% had high scores in both situational and interactional components (Table 1). The mean score for the presumed high risk group was 18.2, for the presumed low-risk group the mean score was 3.3. The extra weighted items affected only 5% of the presumed high risk group: 3.5% were referred because the mother was an adolescent; 1.5% because of known parental history. Thirteen percent of the presumed high risk group required the post-delivery scores to reach the cutoff score.

Interrater Reliability

On the post-delivery observation, overall agreement among the nurses was 84%; on postpartum observation, 96%.

Internal Consistency

On coefficient alpha, the situational part had a reliability of .56 (.70 without special weighting). The post-delivery observation had a reliability of .90, and the postpartum observation had a reliability of .95. The reliability for the overall score was .82 (or .85). Interactional items thus provided the most reliable or consistent discrimination between the presumed high risk and the presumed low risk groups.

The index of predictive association indicated that situational items relating to the characteristics of the infant, medical history, or unemployment, did not contribute to the classification of risk. In the postpartum section, only one item, which related to naming the infant, had a low lambda. Postpartum items were slightly more predictive of risk classification than post-delivery items.

Table 1

BIA - Distribution of Total, Situational and Post-Partum Scores

Score categories	Percent of total (N = 1062)	Percent of presumed high risk (n = 103)
Total score		
Presumed low risk	80.5	
Presumed high risk	19.5	100.0
Excluding post-delivery scores		
High scores on		
1. Situational and post partum	3.6	18.4
2. Situational but not post partum	7.8	39.8
3. Post partum but not situational	4.2	21.4
4. Neither	3.9	20.3
Total high situational[a]	11.4	58.2
Total high post partum[b]	7.8	39.8

Note. Inclusion of post-delivery scores would have introduced three additional scores (high, low, and no score) resulting in a total of 12 categories.

[a] Includes high scores on categories 1 and 2.

[b] Includes high scores on categories 1 and 3.

Predictive Validity

Statistically significant differences, at the .01 level, between the presumed high-risk and presumed low-risk groups, favoring the latter, were obtained on all measures administered at 1 month and on all but the Child Teaching Scale at 1 year (Table 2). This suggested the predictive validity of the BIA for parental performance with respect to responsivity and sensitivity to the infant's needs and cues,

Table 2

Means for One Month and One Year Outcomes for Presumed High Risk and Presumed Low Risk Groups

	Presumed high risk (n = 38)	Presumed low risk (n = 39)
One Month		
HOME	73.08	82.98*
NCAT (Feeding)		
Parent	40.32	43.46*
Child	15.74	18.41*
One Year		
HOME	72.66	86.50*
NCAT (Feeding)		
Parent	40.79	43.89*
Child	18.42	20.54*
NCAT (Teaching)		
Parent	38.24	42.69*
Child	15.89	16.38

*$p < .01$

and opportunities for social, emotional, and cognitive growth of the infant. Correlations between the BIA total score and outcome measures (HOME and NCAF) were stronger for 1 year than for 1 month (Table 3). Interestingly, the situational part of the BIA was more highly correlated with 1 year HOME, and FEEDING (NCAF) scores than either post-delivery or postpartum observations; this was not true for Teaching (NCAT) scores.

DISCUSSION

The Borgess Interaction Assessment was developed as an instrument to screen for newborns in nurturing situations which suggest risk to psycho-social development. The BIA was a reasonable approach for systematizing nurses' observations and referral decisions for early preventive intervention. Observation and review could be incorporated into nursing practice; recording took 10 to 15 minutes.

Unlike the Helfer and Schneider (1975) instrument, it did not require the mother to fill out a form; the nurse's observation and conversation were non-intrusive. The assessment was completed during the hospital stay and did not require subsequent review, as in the NPI. The instrument did not exclude Caesarean births.

Predictive validity of the BIA was strongly indicated by the correlation between the discriminations made at birth and scores on other measures at 1 year which reflected characteristics of the nurturing environment. The higher predictiveness of the situational part would appear to rest primarily on the social support items, in view of the findings in Eyres et al.'s (1980) prospective study that father

Table 3

Correlations between BIA and

One Month and One Year Outcome Scores ($\underline{N}$ = 77)

Age of Infant	Borgess Interaction Assessment			
Measure	Total	Situational	Post-delivery	Post-partum
One Month				
HOME	-.46	-.37	-.40	-.27
NCAF				
Parent	-.28	(-.21)	(-.21)	(-.19)
Child	-.23	(-.21)	(-.15)	(-.13)
One Year				
HOME	-.64	-.54	-.38	-.45
NCAF				
Parent	-.47	-.46	(-.19)	-.32
Child	-.41	-.45	(-.07)	-.28
NCAT				
Parent	-.43	-.30	-.22	-.40
Child	(-.05)	(-.06)	(-.02)	(-.04)

Note. Correlations in parentheses are not significant at the .05 level.

involvement during pregnancy was a strong predictor of IQ, receptive language, and mother's perception of behavior problems at age 4.

The post-delivery scores on the BIA showed lower correlations than the postpartum scores because of the way the instrument was constructed. For one-quarter of the dyads experiencing Caesarean sections, there was no variability on post-delivery scores inasmuch as a standard score of 2 was used when post-delivery observation was not possible. The study of Gray et al. (1977) in Denver found that no increase in predictability occurred by adding postpartum observation to the post-delivery assessment. In the Kalamazoo situation, the nurses in the delivery room were under considerably more pressure than the maternity unit nurses, and found observation and recording more difficult to accomplish. Consequently, the post-delivery observation has been deleted in current use of the BIA in Kalamazoo. Some situational items have also been dropped, based on the internal reliability and consistency data.

It should be noted that the BIA's predictiveness for 12 month scores did not include the child's Teaching score. In other words, the BIA was consistently predictive across measures of the environment, including parental behavior, but was not consistently predictive of the infant's behavior at 12 months.

Why this discrepancy between the patterns for parent-child scores in Feeding and Teaching?

Maternal behavior has been found to be more consistent across situations and across time than is infant behavior (Barnard & Bee, 1982). The feeding situation, being familiar and frequently repeated, might be expected to elicit more congruent interactive behaviors for parent and infant. Conversely, the teaching situation at 12 months, being a new brief experience may elicit more comparable responses from infants regardless of maternal behavior. It is premature to expect significant differences between groups of infants at 12 months on tasks related to development. There seems to be a lack of variability in the results of early developmental testing; differences between children consistent with the characteristics of the nurturing environment are not evident until the second or third year of life (Barnard & Eyres, 1979). The Kalamazoo data indicating that the BIA was not correlated with the child's behavior on the teaching task at 12 months is congruent with Barnard and Eyres' finding that educational status of the mother was not correlated with the child's behavior on the teaching task at 12 months. Similarly,

HOME scores from infancy were predictive of Stanford-Binet scores at 3 years but were only moderately correlated with developmental scales at 12 months (Elardo, Bradley & Caldwell, 1975).

The BIA study did not relate the screening instrument to outcomes in the real world (i.e., evidence of aberrant parenting such as abuse and neglect), nor to assessment of attachment behavior at age 2 or of behavior problems at age 4. This would be desirable for a full exploration of screener predictability. However, funding constraints on the state program mean that this work is unlikely to be accomplished under department or community mental health auspices.

REFERENCES

Ainsworth, M.D.S., Blehar, M.C., Waters, E., & Wall, S. (1978). *The strange situation: Observing patterns of attachment.* Hillsdale, NJ : Erlbaum

Barnard, K.E., & Bee, H.L. (1982). *The assessment of parent-infant interaction by observation of feeding and teaching.* Unpublished manuscript.

Barnard, K.E., & Eyres, S.J. (1979). *Child health assessment, Part 2: The first year of life.* DHEW Pub. No. HRA 79-25. Hyattsville, MD: U.S. Department of Health, Education and Welfare, Public Health Services, Bureau of Health Manpower, Division of Nursing.

Bradley, R.H., & Caldwell, B.M. (1978). Screening the environment. *American Journal of Orthopsychiatry, 48,* 114-130.

Broussard, E.R. (1979). Assessment of the adaptive potential of the mother-infant system: The neonatal perception inventories. *Seminars in Perinatology, 3,* 91-100.

Caldwell, B.M., & Bradley, R.H. (1978). *Manual for the Home Observation for Measurement of the Environment.* Little Rock, AR: University of Arkansas.

Elardo, R., Bradley, R., & Caldwell, B.M. (1975). The relation of infants' home environments to mental test performance from six to thirty-six months: A longitudinal analysis. *Child Development, 46,* 71-76.

Eyres, S., Barnard, K., & Gray, C. (1980). *Child assessment part 3: 2-4 years.* Unpublished manuscript, University of Washington, Seattle.

Fraiberg, S. (1980). *Clinical studies in infant mental health: The first year of life.* New York: Basic Books.

Gray, J.D., Cutler, A., Dean, J.G., & Kempe, C. (1977). Prediction and prevention of child abuse and neglect. *International Journal of Child Abuse and Neglect, 1,* 45-51

Greenspan, S.I., & Lieberman, A.F. (1980). Infants, mothers and their interaction: A quantitative clinical approach to developmental assessment. In S.I. Greenspan & G.H. Pollock (Eds.), *The course of life: Vol. 1, Infancy and early childhood* (pp. 271-312). Washington: U.S. Government Printing Office.

Hayes, W.L. (1973). *Statistics for the social sciences.* New York: Holt, Rinehart and Winston, Inc.

Helfer, R., & Schneider, C. (1975). *Survey on bringing up children.* Unpublished manuscript, Michigan State University, East Lansing.

Lord, F.M., & Novick, M.R. (1968). *Statistical theories of mental test scores.* Reading, MA: Addison-Wesley Publishing Company, Inc.

Sroufe, L.A. (1979). The coherence of individual development. *American Psychologist, 34,* 834-841.

Woods, R.F. (1975). *The infant mental health profile.* Pittsburgh: University of Pittsburgh, Firstborn Project.

The Michigan Association for Infant Mental Health: Historical Context and Contemporary Status

Hiram E. Fitzgerald
Michigan State University

ABSTRACT. The Michigan Association for Infant Mental Health (MAIMH), incorporated in 1977, traces its origins to a clinical training program directed by Selma Fraiberg. However, MAIMH also was a natural reaction to the Zeitgeist of the 1970s which emphasized clinical intervention, applied research, and interdisciplinary collaboration to resolve the problems associated with infancy. MAIMHs activities focus on training and education, professional publications, attention to social issues, continuing education, and promotion of infant mental health organizations internationally. All of MAIMH's activities are guided by its central purpose which is to promote the optimal development of infants and their families.

The Michigan Association for Infant Mental Health (MAIMH) is an interdisciplinary organization whose overriding purpose is to promote the optimal development of infants and their families. Although incorporated in 1977, MAIMH's origins can be traced to 1972 and a small clinical training program at the University of Michigan under the direction of Selma Fraiberg. Fraiberg's training program was, perhaps, a natural outgrowth to the clinical and research interest in infancy that emerged in the 1950s, surged through the '60s, and maintained a high level of intensity to the present. To better understand MAIMH, its history and current status, it may be helpful to place it in its historical context with respect to the

For reprints or information about MAIMH or IAIMH contact Hiram E. Fitzgerald, Ph.D., Executive Officer, MIAMH, Executive Director, IAIMH, Department of Psychology, Psychology Research Building, Michigan State University, East Lansing, MI 48824-1117.

first 2 years of life—that period of human development we now refer to as infancy.

HISTORICAL CONTEXT

The notion that the first 2 years of life is a circumscribed period of human development emerged during the late 19th and 20th centuries. Prior to the 19th century, the term "infant" or "babe" was more typically applied to the elementary school age child (Aries, 1962). The idea that nurturance was an important aspect of development existed as early as the 18th century Enlightenment; the historical period that has been referred to as the "Intrusive Mode of parent-child relations" (DeMause, 1974; cited in Fogel, 1984). Despite recognition of the importance of nurturance for child development, the period of infancy was not viewed as an especially important time in human development nor did "mother love" enjoy the pre-eminence it has achieved in the 20th century (Kagen, Kearsley, & Zelazo, 1978).

Scientific interest in infancy emerged in the 19th century with the publication of baby biographies (Darwin, 1877; Hall, 1896, 1897; Major, 1906; Moore, 1896; Preyer, 1888; Shinn, 1894; Sigismund, 1856), which reflected a broader evolutionary concern for naturalistic description, and with the emergence of psychoanalytic theory which articulated the possibility that infancy was a crucial period in human development. Early in the 20th century, scientific inquiry focused on the infant's sensory, perceptual and motor abilities (Brackbill, 1967). During the World War II era, and for a decade thereafter, attention turned to the effects of environmental influences on the infant's social and emotional development. Seminal publications of the era included those of Ribble (1943) on the "Rights of Infants," Spitz and Wolf (1946) on anaclitic depression, Spitz (1945, 1965) and Goldfarb (1943) on the effects of institutionalization, Freud and Burlingham (1944) on separation, and Bowlby (1952) on maternal care and infant development.

By the 1960s, researchers from a wide variety of disciplines were engaged in the study of infancy. Early in the decade the literature mirrored that of the early 20th century with emphasis on well-controlled laboratory studies of the infant's sensory, perceptual, learning, and attentional abilities. However, results of these investigations challenged the common view that the newborn was a passive recipient of environmental stimulation in possession of a tabula rasa consciousness. At the same time that researchers were discovering the active information processing abilities of the infant, investigators such as Bowlby (1969), Ainsworth (1962), and Fraiberg (1959) were constructing a theme that was to become a major influence on infant studies of the 1970s. Broadly conceived, this theme stressed the importance of the caregiving environment for the infant's affective and social development, encouraged interdisciplinary cooperation, and challenged investigators to apply their research skills to practical problems of everyday life. Thus, in the 1970s attention was given to such issues as infant day care (Caldwell, 1972; Stevenson & Fitzgerald, 1972), home-based developmental intervention (Fitzgerald, 1977; Brajovic, Fitzgerald & Djurdjic, 1978), early educational experiences (Denenberg, 1970), perinatal practices involving mother-infant interaction (Klaus & Kennel, 1976), adolescent pregnancy (McKendry, Walters, & Johnson, 1979), and the cultural context of infant development (Werner, 1972). Selma Fraiberg (1918-1981) emerged from this Zeitgeist as a major spokesperson for the infant mental health movement.

In 1959, Fraiberg's "The Magic Years" focused public attention on the early years of development; in a 15 year period over one million copies of the volume were sold. Less well known to the general public were her publications on blind infants and their families (Fraiberg, 1968), including studies of sensory-motor competence (Fraiberg, Siegal, & Gibson, 1966; Adelson & Fraiberg, 1972, 1974, 1976), mother-infant communication (Fraiberg, 1974; Fraiberg, Smith, & Adelson, 1969), social behavior (Fraiberg, 1970, 1971), and ego development (Fraiberg & Freedman, 1964).

Armed with her vast clinical and research experience, and with grant support from federal and foundation sources, in 1972 Fraiberg established the Child Development Project at the University of Michigan. The project's goal was to develop a home visit psychotherapeutic model of intervention for mother-infant dyads. Fraiberg and her colleagues subsequently contributed to the study of adolescent pregnancy programs (Aradine, Shapiro, & Fraiberg, 1978; Fraiberg, 1971; Shapiro, Fraiberg, & Adelson, 1976), the application of psychoanalytic theory to mother-infant relationships (Fraiberg, Adelson, & Shapiro, 1975) and to the field of social work (Fraiberg, 1978). Her work reflected a commitment to the scientific study of infancy; the integration of psychoanalytic theory with the basic data of child development research; an organismic, dynamic view of the developmental process; and the conviction that to be maximally effective, the study of infancy must be interdisciplinary.

FORMATION OF MAIMH

In 1973, and again in 1974, the Michigan Department of Mental Health persuaded Fraiberg to assign staff to train individuals already working at community mental health agencies as a way of implementing infant mental health services throughout Michigan (Shapiro, Adelson, & Tableman, 1978, 1980, 1982). The 12 individuals enrolled in these two training groups, among the first formally trained community-based infant mental health specialists, were to become the founders of MAIMH.

After completing their formal training, the 12 continued to meet regularly to discuss clinical issues and to plan ways to disseminate the infant mental health perspective to other professionals throughout Michigan (Tableman, 1982a, 1982b; Adelson, Shapiro, & Bennett, 1982). Few could have anticipated the events that were to transpire as a result of those first informal meetings. As a first step in dissemination, a one-day workshop was held, attended by 80 persons. Encouraged by the enthusiastic response to the workshop, in 1976 the group decided to conduct a two-day conference in Ann Arbor. The Michigan Association for Infant Mental Health was created out of the necessity to have a sponsor for the conference. Conference planners hoped for an attendance of 300 to make expenses, but were overwhelmed when nearly 800 registrations poured in from Michigan, other states, and Canada (Tableman, 1982a).

ACTIVITIES OF MAIMH

Now an established organization approaching its 10th anniversary, MAIMH has a stable membership of approximately 300 individuals representing over 13 disciplines, and supports a broad range of clinical, educational, social, and research programs involving infants and their families.

Annual Conference

Building on that initial effort, MAIMH has sponsored an annual conference each year since 1976. Designed to be a continuing education event, the conference features invited speakers from the fields of pediatrics, psychology, social work, nursing, early childhood education, child and family development, and psychiatry, as well as individuals from government agencies responsible for the management of programs affecting infants and their families. In addition, a variety of workshops provide training in the latest approaches to prevention and intervention programming, infant and family assessment, and clinical techniques. Each theme-oriented conference, therefore, serves as a forum for information dissemination about infant mental health work nationally and throughout the state.

Each year at the annual conference, MAIMH honors the memory of Selma Fraiberg by presenting an award in her name to a person or program in the state of Michigan for outstanding contributions to infants and their families.

Publications

During the January 1979 meeting of the Board of Directors it was decided to sponsor a professional journal of international scope consistent with MAIMH's educational mission. In 1980 the first volume of the *Infant Mental Health Journal* was published under the editorship of Jack Stack. The journal publishes articles in four major categories: research, reviews and program descriptions, films and book reviews, and clinical studies. Every volume published to date has included issues dealing with special topics such as fathers and infants, infant assessment, prevention programming, and child abuse.

MAIMH also publishes a quarterly newsletter, *The Infant Crier,* which disseminates information of immediate concern to infant mental health specialists in Michigan. The newsletter allows MAIMH to keep its membership informed about social and legislative issues affecting infants and their families, innovations in program development and implementation, clinical issues, media resources available for parent training and staff development, and other newsworthy items of interest to the membership.

Purpose and Mission

Although MAIMH's bylaws state its purpose as the promotion of optimal development of infants and their families, the rapid growth in membership and the diversity of interests held by the membership required a more detailed statement of MAIMH's policy. This was accomplished during a two-day retreat held in the fall of 1979. The policy statement describes the service sectors expected to have an immediate bearing on the mental health of infants and proposes an explicit plan of action for each service sector. For example:

> MAIMH believes that infants and families need access to health care services in clinics and homes that will optimize and assure normal family development. To this end, MAIMH will encourage the funding and development of public health and medical care services for families and infants.

Ten additional prescriptive statements define MAIMH's mission and provide objectives to guide its activities.

Social Issues

Although MAIMH focuses on issues immediately relevant to mental health, it believes that a narrow definition of mental health is incompatible with a systems view of infant development and family-infant relationships. Moreover, MAIMH recognizes that problems germane to infants and families must be viewed in the context of a broader set of issues relevant to children and families. Therefore, under the direction of Robert Boger, MAIMH's Social Issues Committee chairperson, other organizations concerned with children's issues were invited in 1980 to consider the formation of a coalition to represent the collective interests of all children's and parent-child groups. The Michigan Coalition for Children and Families (MCCF), representing over 20 separate organizations, was the result of that meeting. The MCCF now is recognized as a major advocate for programs in support of children and their families. For example, each year the MCCF prepares a "children's agenda" in response to the proposed state budget allocations for the Departments of Mental Health, Public Health, Education, and Social Services. Thus far the agenda has contributed to legislative support for increased funding of children's programs. The MCCF provides proof that interdisciplinary and multi-interest groups can work constructively to accomplish mutual goals.

Training and Education

In addition to conferences and workshops, MAIMH maintains a library of videotapes and films for use in staff training and/or parent education programs. Most of the videotapes currently available were developed by the Michigan Department of Mental Health. More recent acquisitions were developed by projects sponsored by foundations and Federal grants or by commercial publishing companies. Films are available for rental through the Michigan State University Instructional Media Center, while videotapes are available from MAIMH's central office.

Currently no university-based training program for infant mental health specialists exists in the state of Michigan. To stimulate interest in such programs, MAIMH developed a set of training guidelines in 1983 and disseminated them throughout the state. The guidelines stress training in infant development, infant assessment, research techniques, clinical skills, and program development and evaluation. MAIMH believes that employment opportunities for infant mental health specialists who can undertake clinical and/or educational interventions with multi-problem families will increase during the next decade. Such specialists may be employed directly or under contract by medical care practices, public health clinics, hospitals, protective services agencies, educational institutions, and community agencies. The proposed guidelines, if implemented, would help to ensure a supply of competently trained infant mental health specialists in such agencies and institutions. Copies of the guidelines are available through the MAIMH central office.

IAIMH and Affiliates

The out-of-state representation at the first few annual conferences was so strong that in 1979 the MAIMH Board of Directors voted to sponsor incorporation of the International Association for Infant Mental Health (IAIMH). Within a 4-year span, IAIMH affiliates were established in Texas, Illinois, Iowa, Ontario, Quebec, Mexico, Virginia, northern New England, the Delaware Valley, and North Carolina. Each affiliate is relatively autonomous so that it is free to pursue issues unique to its membership. Members of the IAIMH receive copies of the international newsletter, reduced subscription fees to the *Infant Mental Health Journal*, and reduced rates for the IAIMH annual conference. Perhaps more importantly, the IAIMH serves as a clearinghouse for disseminating information through the network of affiliate associations. Thus, for example, information about a successful clinical intervention program in Texas can be made available to other affiliates through the IAIMH quarterly newsletter more quickly than is possible via the *Infant Mental*

Health Journal. Moreover, since the *IMHJ* is a peer-reviewed journal it is unlikely that descriptions of program innovations would be accepted for publication unless supported by evaluation data.

Local Chapters

During the same 1979 meeting which established the IAIMH, the MAIMH Board also approved the formation of state-level chapters. The local chapter concept expanded rapidly and to date MAIMH has seven geographically restricted chapters, each of which is free to pursue issues of immediate concern at the local level. Thus, chapters in urban areas can deal directly with problems unique to that ecological setting, whereas chapters in more rural regions can deal with their set of unique issues. All chapters embrace MAIMH's overall objectives and work closely with the state association to accomplish MAIMH's mission.

CONCLUSION

Originating from the informal meetings of a small group of individuals who shared a clinical training experience, the Michigan Association for Infant Mental Health has experienced rapid growth. Moreover, it has encouraged formation of similar associations in the United States, Canada, and Mexico. MAIMH is committed to educating professionals and the public about the significance of the early years of human development, the importance of primary prevention, and the necessity of quality programming for infant and family development.

Currently MAIMH is engaged in projects designed to enhance parenting competence, to upgrade education of individuals working directly with infants, to create greater public awareness of the importance of infancy within the spectrum of the human life cycle, to develop guidelines for child abuse prevention and intervention programs, and to upgrade educational opportunities for infant mental health specialists within various disciplines. If changes during the next five years are as rapid as they have been during the past half decade, we have no doubts that the quality of life can be substantially improved for Michigan's infants and their families. We invite clinicians, educators, and researchers from all disciplines to join our efforts to promote the optimal development of infants and their families.

REFERENCES

Adelson, E., & Fraiberg, S. (1972). Mouth and hand in the early development of blind infants. In J. Bosma (Ed.), *Third symposium in oral sensation and perception.* Springfield, IL: Charles C. Thomas.

Adelson, E., & Fraiberg, S. (1974). Gross motor development in infants blind from birth. *Child Development, 45,* 114-126.

Adelson, E., & Fraiberg, S. (1976). Sensory deficit and motor development in infants blind from birth. In Z.S. Jastrzembska (Ed.), *The effects of blindness and other impairments on early development.* Washington D.C.: The American Council for the Blind.

Adelson, E., Shapiro, V., & Bennett, J. (1982). The training of community mental health clinicians as infant specialists. *Infant Mental Health Journal, 3,* 77-83.

Ainsworth, M.D.S. (1962). The effects of maternal deprivation: A review of findings and controversy in the context of research strategy. *Deprivation of maternal care: A reassessment of its effect* (Public Health Papers No. 14, pp. 97-165). Geneva: World Health Organization.

Aradine, C., Shapiro, V., & Fraiberg, S. (1978). Collaborative treatment fosters attachment: Nurse and therapist collaborate in the care of an adolescent high-risk mother pregnant with her second child. *American Journal of Maternal and Child Nursing, 3,*92-98.

Aries, P. (1962). *Centuries of childhood.* New York: Alfred A. Knopf.

Bowlby, J. (1952). *Maternal care and mental health* (Monograph Series Number 2). Geneva: World Health Organization.

Bowlby, J. (1969). *Attachment.* New York: Basic Books.

Brackbill, Y. (Ed.) (1967). *Infancy and early childhood.* New York: The Free Press, p. vi.

Brajovic, C., Fitzgerald, H.E., & Djurdjic, D. (1978). Organizacija kod mentalno retardiranih (Organization of behavior in mental retardates). *Rehabilitacija, 3,* 35-46.

Caldwell, B.M. (1972). What does research teach us about day care: For children under three. *Child Today, 1* (Jan/Feb).

Darwin, C. (1877). A biographical sketch of an infant. *Mind, 2,* 285-294.

Denenberg, V.H. (Ed.). (1970). *Education of the infant and young child.* New York: Academic Press.

DeMause, L. (1974). The evolution of children. In L. DeMause (Ed.), *The history of childhood.* New York: Psychohistory Press.

Fitzgerald, H.E. (1977). Roditelji kod terapeuti dece sa razvojnim disfunkcijama (Parents as therapists for children with developmental disorders). *Psihologija, 10,* 113-120.

Fogel, A. (1984). *Infancy: Infant, family and society.* St. Paul, MN: West Publishing Company.

Fraiberg, S. (1959). *The magic years.* New York: Charles Scribner's Sons.

Fraiberg, S. (1968). Parallel and divergent patterns in blind and sighted infants. *Psychoanalytic study of the child* (Vol. 23). New York: International Universities Press.

Fraiberg, S. (1970). Smiling and stranger reaction in blind infants. In J. Hellmuth (Ed.), *The exceptional infant* (Vol 2). New York: Brunner/Mazel.

Fraiberg, S. (1971). Intervention in infancy. *Journal of American Academy of Child Psychiatry, 10,* 381-405.

Fraiberg, S. (1974). Blind infants and their mothers: An examination of the sign system. In M. Lewis & L.A. Rosenblum (Eds.), *The effect of the infant on its caregiver.* New York: Wiley-Interscience.

Fraiberg, S. (1978). Psychoanalysis and social work: A reexamination of the issues. *Smith College Studies in Social Work, 48,* 87-106.

Fraiberg, S., Adelson, E., & Shapiro, V. (1975). Ghosts in the nursery: A psychoanalytic approach to the problems of impaired infant-mother relationships. *Journal of the American Academy of Child Psychiatry, 14,* 387-421.

Fraiberg, S., & Freedman, D. (1964). Studies in the ego development of the congenitally blind child. *Psychoanalytic study of the child* (Vol 21). New York: International Universities Press.

Fraiberg, S., Siegal, B., & Gibson, R. (1966). The role of sound in the search behavior of a blind infant. *Psychoanalytic study of the child* (Vol 21). New York: International Universities Press.

Fraiberg, S., Smith, M., & Adelson, E. (1969). An educational program for blind infants. *Journal of Special Educational, 3,* 121-139.

Freud, A., & Burlingham, D. (1944). *Infants without families.* New York: International Universities Press.

Goldfarb, W. (1943). Infant rearing and problem behavior. *American Journal of Orthopsychiatry, 13,* 249-365.

Hall, W.S. (1896). The first five hundred days of a child's life. *The Child Study Monthly, 2,* 330-342, 394-407.

Hall, W.S. (1897). The first five hundred days of a child's life. *The Child Study Monthly, 2,* 458-473, 522-537.

Kagen, J., Kearsley, R.B., & Zelazo, P.R. (1978). *Infancy: Its place in human development.* Cambridge, MA: Harvard University Press.

Klaus, M.H., & Kennell, J.H. (1976). *Maternal-infant bonding.* St. Louis: Mosby.

Major, D.R., (1906). *First steps in mental growth.* New York: MacMillan.

McKendry, J.C., Walters, L.H. & Johnson, C. (1979). Adolescent pregnancy: A review of the literature. *The Family Coordinator, 28,* 17-28.

Moore, K.C. (1896). *Mental development of a child.* New York: MacMillan.

Preyer, W. (1888). *The mind of the child, Part I: The senses and the will* (2nd ed., H.W. Bram, Trans.), New York: D. Appleton & Company.

Ribble, M. (1943). *The rights of infants.* New York: Columbia University Press.

Shapiro, V., Adelson, E., & Tableman, B. (1978). A model for the introduction of infant mental health services to community mental health agencies. *Journal of the American Academy of Child Psychiatry, 17,* 283-355.

Shapiro, V., Adelson, E., & Tableman, B. (1980). Beginning at the beginning: The introduction of mental health services to community mental health. In S. Fraiberg (Ed.), *Clinical studies in infant mental health: The first year of life.* New York: Basic Books.

Shapiro, V., Adelson, E., & Tableman, B. (Eds.). (1982). The introduction of infant mental health services in Michigan. *Infant Mental Health Journal, 3,* 69-141.

Shapiro, V., Fraiberg, S., & Adelson, E. (1976). Infant parent psychotherapy on behalf of a child in a critical nutritional state. *Psychoanalytic study of the child* (Vol. 31). New York: International Universities Press.

Shinn, M.W. (1894). *Notes on the development of a child.* Berkeley: University of California Press.

Sigismund, B. (1856) *Kind and welt: Die funt esten perioden des kindesalters.* Braunschweig: Viewegund sohn.

Spitz, R.A. (1945). Hospitalism. *Psychoanalytic study of the child* (Vol. 1). New York: International Universities Press.

Spitz, R.A. (1965). *The first year of life.* New York: International Universities Press.

Spitz, R.A., & Wolf, K.W. (1946). The smiling response: A contribution to the ontogenesis of social relations. *Genetic Psychology Monographs, 34,* 57-125.

Stevenson, M. B., & Fitzgerald, H.E. (1972). Standards for infant day care in the United States and Canada. *Child Care Quarterly, 1,* 89-111.

Tableman, B. (1982a). Infant mental health: A new frontier. *Infant Mental Health Journal, 3,* 72-76.

Tableman, B. (1982b). What happened after training: The development of infant mental health services. *Infant Mental Health Journal, 3,* 84-89.

Werner, E.E. (1972). Infants around the world: Cross cultural studies of psychomotor development from birth to two years. *Journal of Cross-cultural Psychology, 3,* 111-134.

A Parent Education Project for Low-Income Families

Michael Mischley
E. Webb Stacy, Jr.
Lynne Mischley
David Dush
Midland-Gladwin Community Mental Health Services Board

ABSTRACT. The impact of the Midland Parent Education Project on a low-income population with preschool children was assessed. The program consisted of a five-session structured multimodal group program supplemented by two home visits and a concurrent nursery program. Financial incentives were provided for attendance. A nonequivalent control group design was used, with a pretest, posttest, and extended posttest for the experimental group and a pretest and extended posttest for the control group. There were gains in the experimental group's parenting skills level (both absolutely, and relative to the control group) during the training period and on follow-up. The children's social competency increased during the training period for the experimental (but not the control) group, and continued to increase for 6 months following the training event when age effects were considered. Children's social competency scores were correlated with parents' scores on specific parenting skills.

Research evidence suggests a crucial role for family environment and parenting styles in the adjustment of children (Coopersmith, 1967; Martin, 1975; Minuchin, 1974; Mischler & Waxler, 1968; Patterson, 1982; Rohner, 1975). Studies have focused on the effect of the family on self-esteem, aggression, neurotic and behavioral disorders, psychosomatic problems, and academic problems. In ad-

---

The project was originally developed under funding from the U.S. Office of Economic Opportunity, Grant No. 50572. The secondary analysis of the relationship between social competency and parenting skills was undertaken by Carolyn L. Feis of the Michigan Department of Mental Health.

Reprints are available from the senior author, Midland Psychological Consultants, P.C., 4908 Mac Court, Midland, MI 48640.

dition, it appears that social class differences in parenting styles seem to render children of low-income families more vulnerable to problems with emotional, social, and cognitive development (Chilman, 1965; Escalona, 1981; Martin, 1975). Studies making class comparisons indicate that lower socioeconomic parents "were more likely to use ridicule, shouting, or physical punishment with their children. They tended to use power assertive disciplinary techniques and a minimum of verbal give-and-take" (Alvey, 1981, p. 29). Furthermore, these influences are evident very early in life (Escalona, 1981; White, Kabin, & Attanucci, 1979).

Despite the importance of the family to the psychosocial growth of children, in our society parenting and family management skills are not expected to be taught. A successful educational effort with low-income families is particularly difficult in view of such characteristics as lack of success in school, limited income, and in many, rural isolation. A summary (Lockman & Brown, 1980) of the relationship between participant demographic variables and outcome in parent education groups found reports of decreased problem behaviors and increased appropriate behaviors in children to be positively correlated with parents' educational level (Saddler, Seyden, Howe, & Kaminsky, 1976) and parents' income (Rinn, Vernon, & Wise, 1975). In addition, Rinn and his associates found that parents who dropped out of their parent training groups tended to have lower incomes.

Based on this research data and a survey indicating that preschool children were a population underserved by the Midland-Gladwin Community Mental Health Services, a parent education program was undertaken by the agency. The program was a primary prevention project aimed at promoting healthy child development in low-income families with preschool children—a high risk portion of the underserved preschool population.

The present study was designed to evaluate the effectiveness of a five-session structured, multimodel parent education program (Mischley, Mischley, & Ingold, 1983) supplemented by two home visits and a concurrent nursery program, offered to low-income families with preschool children by a community mental health center.

It was hypothesized that (a) parents would show significant increases in parenting skill levels following training and maintain their skills on follow-up, and that (b) the preschool children in the family would show significant increases in social competency.

METHOD

Participants

All of the families met two eligibility requirements: (a) the family had to be classified as "low-income," with an annual income of less than $8,500 for two persons plus $750 for each additional dependent in the family; and (b) the family must also have had at least one child older than 18 months, but not having started kindergarten, although they may have had other children outside the age group. Characteristics of the experimental and control groups are defined in Table 1.

Experimental and control groups were selected in the same manner although each came from a different but adjacent county. A brochure, a letter to parents, and a return postcard were developed to inform referring persons and potential families of the program. The return postcards initiated the contacts with interested families. Primary community service agencies, physicians, ministers, and other possible referral sources were informed about the program, given the brochures, letters, and postcards, and periodically contacted about potential referrals or questions they might have.

Table 1

Participants

	Experimental		Control	
	N	%	N	%
Families	42		30	
Female Parents	42	100	30	100
Male Parents	11	26	12	40
Boys	27	64	17	56
Girls	27	64	19	63
Two Children Families	12	29	6	20
Average Age (months)	36		38	

Another recruitment method was a poster in the lobbies of primary service agencies. The poster contained postcards to be filled out by interested parents. Some agencies provided lists of families with young children and those families were sent the brochure and contacted by telephone when possible.

From the time of enrollment to actually attending the program, the attrition rate was approximately 15%. This was due to many factors, such as moving, changing jobs, enrollment in adult education, or other time conflicts. When the time and day for each program was set, it was based on the best possible time for all families involved. Those who could not attend were offered other opportunities in later groups. Of those families who attended one or more sessions, only 5% did not complete the series. This dropout rate was also due to a variety of reasons such as illness, loss of interest, and job changes. The relatively low dropout rates were influenced by offering make-up sessions to parents who had to unavoidably miss a session. As a result, parents included in the analyses did participate in all sessions.

Program

The overall program consisted of five group training sessions for parents, an incentive program for attendance, two home visits, and a nursery program (see Mischley et al., 1983, for an extended manual). The selection and design of the program curriculum were tailored to the anticipated parenting skill deficits of low-income populations as described above. The program is outlined below.

Educational series. The parent group training approach was chosen for its supportive interpersonal features. The educational series had five 2-hour group training modules. Each module emphasized concrete skills that could be practiced in the session rather than reading and/or lecture formats. Teaching several types of parenting techniques appeared to be the most effective means of helping parents cope with a wide range of problems. The skills chosen were seen as positive additions or alternatives to typical lower socioeconomic parenting styles. One previous uncontrolled study (Saddler et al., 1976) of a structured parent group combining two parenting modalities (communication and behavior management) did find that children decreased problem behaviors, increased their compliance, and that parents became more positively reinforcing following training. The first module focused on play experiences which were inexpensive, available to most households, and involved interaction with the parent. The second module focused on listening and problem-solving skills and was derived from Gordon (1970). The third module centered on behavior management techniques, such as positive reinforcement, mild social punishment, ignoring, and time out. This material was adapted from *Effective Parents/ Responsible Children* (Eimers & Aitchison, 1977). The fourth module covered building positive strengths—self-concept, responsibility taking, and independence. It was based on work emphasizing the importance of building positive coping skills (Kangas & Solomon, 1975). The fifth module was aimed at helping parents to determine which approach to use with their children in different situations.

Financial incentive. A financial incentive system contingent on attendance was integral to the program. Previous studies had suggested the necessity and usefulness of employing monetary contingencies in training parents (Cone & Sloop, 1974; Rinn et al., 1975). Payment was $5.00 for a single parent and $7.00 for a couple for each session attended and a $5.00 per person bonus for attending all sessions. Parents missing a session received a reduced incentive of $3.50 a single person and $5.00 a couple for attending a make-up session. For many families this money covered gas expenses but also was designed to motivate interest in participating.

Home visits. The group educational program was supplemented by two home visits by a trained parent educator to individualize instruction and to assist parents in generalizing skills learned in the classroom to the actual home emvironment. Previous studies had suggested that parents did not always generalize skills learned in training (Embry, 1981; Wahler, 1980). One home visit occurred midway through the program and the other after completion of the program. In the home visits, emphasis was placed on reviewing skills taught in group sessions and covering application in specific situations.

Nursery program. The nursery school experience was incorporated to provide a childcare arrangement while parents attended group sessions, a brief positive group experience for the children, and a means of identifying problem behaviors to discuss in home visits. The nursery program consisted of planned gross and fine motor activities.

Design

It was not politically feasible to randomly assign subjects to treatment and no-treatment control conditions since the demonstration project was part of ongoing community service efforts. Consequently, a nonequivalent control group design was employed: all referrals within one of the two counties served by the agency were admitted to the experimental treatment group while referrals in the other adjacent county were assigned to a delayed treatment control group that was not offered services until the end of the study. Due to limited resources in the area, it was unlikely that control group subjects had available any other parenting services during the delay period. This design provided an untreated comparison group against which the treatment effects can be contrasted, but results should be viewed in light of the threats to internal and external validity that attend the nonequivalent control group design (Campbell & Stanley, 1963), limiting the ability to make confident causal inferences.

There was some assurance of the initial equivalence of the groups since the admission criteria kept both groups similar in income level. Table 1 also illustrates that other characteristics of participants were similar across groups. The largest differences were the greater proportion of male parents in the control group and of families with two preschool children in the experimental group. We cannot be certain of the importance of these differences, but experience suggests that the increased parental involvement would, if anything, favor the control group.

Both groups were pretested and tested again 7 1/2 months later. The experimental group was also tested 6 weeks after the pretest to measure the immediate impact of the intervention. All participants included in the analyses completed all testing sessions. The repeated testing itself is unlikely to have substantially influenced outcome: a separate study of this program, with identical tests and similar randomly assigned participants in various sequences of repeated testing, found no evidence of bias introduced by pretesting or repeated posttests (Dush & Stacy, 1984).

Instruments

Three instruments were used at each testing to measure program effects. The first was the CPSCS, California Preschool Social Competency Scale (Levine, Elzey, & Lewis, 1969). The CPSCS was a

30 item rating scale designed to assess the social competency of preschoolers, tapping adequacy of interpersonal behavior, assumption of a social responsibility, ability to make transitions and follow instructions, and emergence of independence. The test was normed on a sample of 800 children, aged 2 to 5, from diverse geographical regions and both high and low sociological levels as gauged by fathers' occupational level. It claimed high internal consistency (split-half reliabilities ranging from .90 to .98) and respectable interrater reliabilities ranging from .75 to .86.

The CPSCS was standardized on ratings of teachers and other school personnel, but it was designed to be rated by anyone familiar enough with the child's behavior to be able to accurately respond to the 30 descriptive behavioral items. The present study used parents as raters. A comparison of parent and teacher ratings at the end of the intervention established the reliability of parent ratings, therefore, parent ratings were used exclusively. Because of the low verbal skills of some participants, minor wording changes were made to simplify some items. The changes were minimal, but caution is nonetheless due in interpreting the exact equivalence of present CPSCS scores to those of the normative data.

The second type of instrument was a behavioral observation checklist of parenting skills in structured role playing tasks, patterned after the approach of Eimers and Aitchison (1977), tailored to assess the types of skills taught. The checklists drew heavily on the content of Sessions 2 (listening and problem solving) and 3 (behavioral management techniques). For example, a checklist for the behavioral technique of "praise" used the role play:

> Your daughter Mary just picked up her toys without being asked. I will play your daughter and please show me how you would praise her.

The score for this task was produced by summing the number of the following items that were observed in the parent's response:

1. looks at Mary,
2. physical proximity (within 3 feet),
3. smiles,
4. non-verbal gestures of approval (touch, hold, hug, or kiss),
5. 5 second latency or less,
6. verbally positive,
7. praise behavior, not child.

A total of six checklists (Praise, Ignoring, Active Listening, Time Out, Mild Social Punishment, and Problem Solving) were summed to produce a total score ranging from 0 to a maximum of 60. All checklists were described in further detail elsewhere (Mischley et al., 1983).

The final instrument was the HOME, Home Observation for Measurement of the Environment (Caldwell & Bradley, 1978), assessing the overall adequacy of the home environment provided by both parents. Unfortunately, interrater reliability problems with the HOME compromised the usefulness of this instrument so the data were not included in the analysis.

RESULTS

Only data provided by mothers was used in the analysis. The pretest and posttest data were analyzed in a 2 (group) by 2 (assessments) repeated measures analysis of variance (ANOVA). Notwithstanding possible inequivalencies of the groups at the outset, the hypothesized treatment effects were represented by the group by assessment ANOVA interaction term.

Social Competency

Table 2 shows that the experimental group was not significantly different from the control group on the CPSCS at pretest ($p > .05$). There was a differential change across groups, however, producing significant group by assessment interaction, $F\ (1,88) = 8.0$, $p < .01$. Indeed, while the experimental group began at a level comparable to the control group, their posttest performance exceeded that of the control group, $F\ (1,88) = 43.6$, $p < .001$. This represented a significant gain for the experimental group ($p < .001$), but no significant change over time for the controls. This gain for the experimental group was evident immediately after completion, and had increased further at follow-up testing.

The "meaningfulness" of this change can be gauged by viewing the various group means as scores representative of "typical" children in the program, and comparing their scores to normative data for the CPSCS. For illustrative purposes, the collapsed norms for all children in the 3-year old CPSCS sample were referenced. Thus, the "typical" child in the experimental group began at a score

Table 2

Mean Scores for Experimentals and Controls on Outcome Measures

Outcome Variable	Experimental Group	Control Group
CPSCS		
Pretest	67.2	75.4
Immediate Posttest	76.1	-
Follow-up	85.6*	70.1
Behavioral Checklist		
Pretest	15.3*	27.6
Immediate Posttest	36.1	-
Follow-up	34.4*	28.6

*p<.001.

which would fall at the 23rd percentile and at follow-up performed at the 66th percentile relative to other boys or the 58th percentile relative to other girls. These gains were actually sufficient to place follow-up performance of the experimental group above average levels of the norm sample of children of high occupational level families, while they initially performed below the 15th percentile compared to this advantaged reference group. In contrast, the control group actually declined by over 10 percentile points. This decline was not significant, and may simply reflect random fluctuation.

Parenting Skills

The total score from the role-play behavior checklists (Table 2) revealed that the experimental group began lower than the control group, F (1,70) = 65.5, $p < .001$; changed differentially,

$F(1,70) = 141.3$, $p < .001$; and ended up at follow-up significantly higher than performance of the control group, $F(1,70) = 80.0$, $p < .001$). This represents a significant gain for the experimental group ($p < .001$), but no significant change over time for controls. The gain for the experimental group was evident at immediate posttest and did not diminish significantly across the time of follow-up.

Relationships Between Social Competency and Parenting Skills

A secondary analysis was undertaken to determine which techniques of parenting skills were related to changes in social competency in children. A simple regression with pairwise deletion of missing data was used in three different combinations. Regression equations were run with mothers only, fathers only, and the average of both parents (where data were available for only the mother, her score was used as the average). All data were based on change scores from pretest to termination (treatment condition was included as a dummy variable).

The parenting techniques of mothers which were found to be most predictive of change in social competency included Ignoring, Active Listening (negative Beta weight), Time Out (negative), and Mild Social Punishment. For fathers, Problem Solving was the most predictive parenting technique. When the scores for both parents were combined (Table 3), Ignoring, Time Out (negative), and Active Listening (negative) were most predictive of changes in social competence of the children. The pattern of results for the average parent scores resembles that of mothers only because in over two-thirds of the cases, there were data on mothers only.

DISCUSSION

Notwithstanding the limitations of design and measurement, the results suggested that (a) there were major gains in parenting skills and child social competency for treated subjects but not for controls; (b) these effects were evident immediately after participation, and persisted or increased across the additional follow-up period; (c) with reference to at least the CPSCS, these gains were of sufficient magnitude to raise the group performance from a clearly disadvantaged level to an average level; and (d) there are identifiable parenting changes which were predictive of improvement in the social competency of children.

Table 3

Regression of Childrens' Social Competency Change Scores with Parents' Module Change Scores, Averaged, Pretest to Termination

Variable	B	$F(7, 50)$
Active Listening	-1.19	4.11*
Problem Solving	0.18	0.04
Mild Social Punishment	0.67	2.22
Ignoring	2.29	9.23**
Time Out	-1.49	6.95*
Praise	1.32	1.97
Condition (Dummy)	0.	

Note. The constant, which represents the Y-intercept, is equal to 4.22. The proportion of variance accounted for by the variables is 30%: $R^2 = .30$. $F(7, 50) = 3.06^{**}$, showing that the variables listed are statistically related to the social competency change scores.

$^{*}p < .05$. $^{**}p < .01$.

Interestingly, Bartlett (1932) suggested that most material newly learned in a short period of time is forgotten within 6 months unless it is in repeated use. Thus, the present data imply that the parents did use and retain the skills taught in the program.

One question that must be raised is why this parenting program was successful when other studies have found that "even if parents and children exhibited significant improvements at the end of training, they did not always maintain those skills over time or generalize those skills to other settings" (Embry, 1981, p.18). An attractive hypothesis is that novel features of the present program facilitated attendance and learning. The program was designed to be well suited to characteristics of the target population. The mid-program and post-program home visits individualized and encouraged using the skills taught within the home setting. Make-up sessions assured that all participants received the "full treatment." The low attrition rate compared to many studies of low SES recipients may also have been partly a function of the financial incentive program and the extensive contact for the in-home assessments. Dush and Stacy (1984) found that recipients randomly assigned to be pretested and posttested had only 1/3 the dropout rate of those who received posttest only. Finally, the approach was family oriented and multimodal—features which may provide a broader more flexible intervention than traditional approaches.

These conclusions must, for the present, be viewed as tentative, given methodological limitations. Further research and replication should incorporate a true experimental design permitting stronger causal inference and nonreactive measures that would be less vulnerable to demand, experimenter bias, or other distortions. It would also be important for further studies to consider (a) longer term follow-up, including academic performance and emotional development of the children; (b) a broad array of outcome variables exploring the possible areas of program impact; and (c) analysis of the components of the program to determine the "active" ingredients and the optimal array and delivery of treatment elements. It is particularly important to isolate the contribution of the nursery school experience and other innovative features of the program.

In summary, there was evidence in the pretest data that a brief educational prevention program of five group sessions, two individualized home sessions, and a concurrent nursery experience resulted in significant gains for the experimental group of parents and children. Importantly, these benefits appeared to persist or perhaps grow over time. Given the magnitude of impact at a rather modest expenditure of effort, the program's approach clearly warrants replication and further study.

REFERENCE NOTE

1. Further analysis of parenting skills measures and their relationship to child social competency are reported in: Dush, D.M. (1984). *Evaluation update: Parent Education Program, Preschool Series.* Technical report: Midland-Gladwin Community Mental Health Services. The report can be obtained from the senior author

REFERENCES

Alvey, K. (1981). *The enhancement of parenting: An analysis of parent training programs.* Studio City, CA: CICC.

Bartlett, F. C. (1932). *Remembering.* Cambridge, England: Cambridge University Press.

Caldwell, B.M., & Bradley, R.H. (1978). *Manual for the Home Observation for Measurement of the Environment.* Little Rock, AR: University of Arkansas.

Campbell, D.H., & Stanley, J.C. (1963). *Experimental and quasi-experimental designs for research.* Chicago: Rand-McNally.

Chilman, C.S. (1965). Childrearing and family life patterns of the very poor. *Welfare in Review, 3,* 9-11.

Cone, J.D., & Sloop, E.W. (1974). Parents as agents of change. In A. Jacobs & W.W. Spradlen (Eds.), *The group as agent of change.* New York: Behavioral Publications.

Coopersmith, S. (1967). *The antecedents of self-esteem.* San Francisco: W.H. Freeman and Co.

Dush, D.M., & Stacey, E.W., Jr. (1984). *Pretesting enhancement of parent compliance in a prevention program for high-risk children.* Unpublished manuscript.

Eimers, R., & Aitchison, R. (1977). *Effective parents/responsible children.* New York: McGraw-Hill.

Embry, L. (1981). *Two emerging models of parent training: General and problem-specific.* Paper presented at First Annual Symposium of Applied Behavioral Analysis in Education, Mexico City.

Escalona, S. (1981). Infant day care: A social and psychological perspective on mental health implications. *Infant Mental Health Journal, 2,* 4-17.

Gordon, T. (1970). *P.E.T.: Parent effectiveness training.* New York: Weyden.

Kangas, J., & Solomon, G. (1975). *The psychology of strength.* Englewood Cliffs: Prentice Hall.

Levine, S., Elzey, F.F., & Lewis, M. (1969). *California Preschool Social Competency Scale manual.* Palo Alto: Consulting Psychologists Press.

Lockman, J., & Brown, M. (1980). Evaluation of dropout clients and of perceived usefulness of a parent education program. *Journal of Community Psychology, 8,* 132-139.

Martin, B. (1975). Child-parent relations. In F. Horowitz (Ed.), *Review of child development research* (Vol. 4). Chicago: University of Chicago Press.

Minuchin, S. (1974). *Families and family therapy.* Cambridge, MA: Harvard University Press.

Mischler, E., & Waxler, N. (1968). *Interaction in families: An experimental study of family processes and schizophrenia.* New York: John Wiley & Sons.

Mischley, M., Mischley, L., & Ingold, B. (1983). *Parent education for low income families with young children.* Lansing, MI: Michigan Department of Mental Health.

Patterson, G.R. (1982). *Coercive family process.* Eugene: Castalia Publishing Co.

Rinn R.C., Vernon, J.C., & Wise, M.J. (1975). Training parents of behaviorally disordered children in groups: A three years' program evaluation. *Behavior Therapy, 6,* 378-387.

Rohner, R.P. (1975). *They love me, they love me not: A worldwide study of the effects of parental acceptance and rejection.* New Haven: HRAF Press.

Saddler, D.W., Seyden, T., Howe, B., & Kaminsky, T. (1976). An evaluation of groups for parents: A standarized format encompassing behavior modification and humanistic methods. *Journal of Community Psychology, 4,*157-163.

Wahler, R.G. (1980). The insular mother: Her problems in parent child treatment. *Journal of Applied Behavior Analysis, 13,* 23-39.

White, B.L., Kaban, B., & Attanucci, J. (1979). *The origins of human competence.* Lexington, MA: Lexington Books.

Training Preschool Children in Interpersonal Cognitive Problem-Solving Skills: A Replication

Carolyn L. Feis
Michigan Department of Mental Health

Craig Simons
Grand Rapids Catholic Social Services

ABSTRACT. Interpersonal Cognitive Problem-Solving training, developed to teach children how (rather than what) to think and therefore how to solve their own interpersonal problems, was used in a study over three years conducted in Newaygo County, Michigan to evaluate its impact on low-income preschool children. Overall, trained children improved in both their ability to solve interpersonal problems, and in their classroom behavior. Control children showed no such systematic improvement. The relationships between problem-solving ability and classroom behavior were observed directly and found to be positively related. The findings of these three studies indicate that interpersonal problem-solving training is useful with low-income, rural children.

One of the few prevention initiatives that has been extensively evaluated is Interpersonal Cognitive Problem-Solving training (ICPS) developed by Myrna Shure (Spivack & Shure, 1974). Recognized in the literature as a major prevention strategy (Cowen, 1977), ICPS received the Lela Rowland prevention award from the National Mental Health Association in 1983. As the first round of pilot demonstration projects was being developed in Michigan,

---

Analyses were undertaken by William L. Redmon and Pamela Luttig (Years 1 and 2) and Accelerative Education Associates (Year 3).

Reprints may be obtained from Carolyn L. Feis, Prevention and Demonstration Projects, Michigan Department of Mental Health, Lewis Cass Building, Lansing, MI 48926.

ICPS was selected for replication and evaluation as a community service model.

ICPS grew out of Spivack's observation, validated by subsequent research, that the ability to problem solve distinguishes normal individuals from those exhibiting behavioral and emotional problems (Shure & Spivack, 1980, 1982). The ability to generate alternative solutions was found to mediate behavior in young children, while the ability to conceptualize causes and consequences was more significant in adults (Spivack, Platt, & Shure, 1976).

ICPS was developed as a training program for young children to teach them not what to think but rather how to think so that they can solve their own interpersonal problems. Specifically, the program was designed to reduce maladaptive behavior and to foster positive mental health in both normal and high-risk children by building coping strategies through interpersonal skill development (Shure & Spivack, 1982).

Shure and Spivack evaluated the impact of training inner city children in ICPS at both the preschool and the kindergarten level (Shure, 1981; Shure & Spivack, 1979, 1980, 1982). In a carefully sequenced research effort, they concluded that mastery of problem-solving skills reduces aberrant behavior, maintains these improvements over time, and prevents behavioral problems that could arise when children are confronted by the demands of primary grades. In terms of the amount of training needed, they found that one training program, whether in preschool or kindergarten, was sufficient for behavioral adjustment.

ICPS is considered to be an antecedent to adjustment because of the direct relationship observed between improvement in problem-solving skills and behavior (Shure, 1982). For both the preschool and kindergarten trained children, problem-solving skills increased from pre- to posttesting significantly more than for controls, independent of IQ (Shure, 1982; Shure & Spivack, 1979). Behaviorally, impulsive children became less demanding and impatient while inhibited children became more outgoing and sociable. Those who improved behaviorally were significantly more likely to improve in their problem-solving skills than were those who did not improve behaviorally.

Preschool controls who were behind at kindergarten did not catch up to trained children 6 months or 1 year later despite natural developmental gains. Shure (1982) further found that children who did not exhibit behavioral problems at the preschool level and who were not trained showed significantly more behavior problems at kindergarten than did similar children who were trained. This demonstrates further the preventive effects of ICPS training.

In a study of children from a private preschool, Ridley and Vaughn (1982) found that trained children showed significantly more improvement in problem solving than did controls immediately after training and 3 months later.

While some studies appear to find conflicting results (Gillespie, Durlak, & Sherman, 1982; Rickel & Burgio, 1982), this may reflect the way in which training was replicated. It appears important that teachers do the training, rather than outsiders, so that skills can be generalized beyond the training lessons. Further, the effects are limited without the use of dialoguing as real problem situations occur.

The replication of ICPS in Michigan was undertaken as a pilot demonstration project in a rural Headstart program serving predominantly white children in Newaygo County. The project was designed to assess the generalizability of ICPS effects from the inner city children evaluated by Shure to the rural children targeted in this study. The purpose was to see if ICPS would work in a community field setting in Michigan.

The study required 3 years to collect data on both skills acquisition and behavioral change due to problems encountered with the behavioral measure in the initial years. The behavioral measure used the first year was found to be unreliable. Therefore during the second year, an effort was made to locate a reliable, standardized measure of behavioral change. The training was continued in order to maintain the teacher's skill at using ICPS. A new behavioral measure was included the third year.

METHOD

Subjects

Participants in all three years (1978, 1979, 1980) were low-income preschool children enrolled in the Newaygo Headstart program. Classrooms were randomly assigned to experimental and control groups and all children were participants. In the first year, complete data was obtained for 15 students in three experimental classrooms who received the problem-solving training and 14 students in two control classrooms who received no intervention. In the second year, there were complete data at the end of the year for 15 children from one classroom in each treatment condition. In the third year, 17 children in the classroom receiving the problem-solving training, and 18 children in the control classroom had complete data.

Intervention

The Newaygo project used Shure and Spivack's (1974/1978) kindergarten script in training teachers to interact with the children (Shure, 1976). The daily dialogues and games lasted about 20 minutes each and took about three months to complete (Spivack & Shure, 1974). Dialoguing, however, was continued after the scripts had been completed.

The program was divided into two phases. The first phase taught prerequisite skills necessary for problem solving. First, vocabulary concepts such as "and-or," "same-diferent," "happy-sad," and "not" were presented in playful scripts. Secondly, identification of feelings and clarification of emotions was taught. The second phase of the training developed problem-solving skills directly. Students were taught to think of multiple solutions and then to evaluate them on their potential consequences. They were encouraged to use creative problem solving in relation to behavioral or interpersonal issues.

A significant component of the training process was dialoguing. Teachers were encouraged to use the problem-solving sequence whenever interpersonal conflict occurred. This process taught children to use ICPS when confronted with real-life problems. It also created a consistency between the formal lessons and life events by applying the skills learned in the training sessions across various problem situations (Shure, 1981, 1982; Shure & Spivack, 1982).

Instruments

Preschool Interpersonal Problem-Solving Test (PIPS). The instrument, developed by Spivack and Shure (1974), was designed to measure preschoolers' ability to solve interpersonal problems. The PIPS test had two parts. The first part presented a series of stories describing problems between peers. In each case there was conflict over competing desires, i.e., one child wanted to play with a toy that another child was using. The child was then asked how he/she would act if faced with that situation. The second part involved stories depicting situations in which a child had done something that had made his/her mother angry. The child was then asked to think about ways to avoid the mother's anger.

The procedure was designed to elicit as many different solutions as possible from each child. The instructions were worded so as to encourage the child to give a different solution to each story that was presented. In part 1, the children were presented with at least seven similar peer-toy situations. If unique solutions were given to each of the seven stories, the tester continued until no new solutions were offered. In part 2, the same procedure was followed, except that a minimum of five mother's potential anger stories were provided. After the tester asked the first question, three probes were offered, allowing the child four opportunities to provide solutions to each situation.

The PIPS yielded two scores. The number of new relevant solutions to the problem were recorded as Solutions. The number of Solution Categories (i.e., tricks, seeking authority intervention, negotiating, or manipulation) were also recorded. This instrument was used all three years as a measure of problem-solving ability.

Teacher's Behavior Rating Scale. This non-standardized nine point scale, developed by program staff to measure changes in interpersonal behavior as a result of the progam, was used in the first year of the study.

Preschool Behavioral Questionnaire (PBQ). The scale measured the extent to which children demonstrated problem behavior suggestive of the emergence of emotional problems (Behar & Stringfield, 1974). Items scored from 0 to 2 comprised three subscales: (a) hostile/aggressive, (b) anxious, and (c) hyperactivity/distractable and a total score. This instrument was used in the third year of the study.

Procedure

In each of the 3 years of the study, a pre-post control-experimental group design was used. The prevention coordinator, a psychologist, trained teachers and aides in a one-day session prior to the start of the program. This training included the structuring of class time so that teachers would be organized in such a way as to accommodate ICPS. Approximately 1 month and 4 months later, two

3-hour in-service training sessions were held to subsequently reinforce the training and address problems. In addition, weekly consultation was provided both in and outside the classroom.

ICPS was used by each of the preschool teachers and aides as part of the usual program. Pretest ratings were all done at the beginning of the school year. The first 2 years of the study posttested at the end of the school year, while the third year posttested immediately after training was completed (10 weeks). In each year, the PIPS was administered by trained personnel from outside the school and the behavior ratings were completed by each of the teachers, who were not blind as to the treatment conditions of the children.

RESULTS

Year 1

Demographic comparisons of participants revealed that trained children were older than control group children, $\chi^2(3) = 8.30$, $p < .05$. Other demographic variables showed no significant differences, i.e., sex, percent attendance, sibling involvement, family marital status, and classroom size.

PIPS. A two-factor analysis of variance revealed that the study and control groups were not significantly different in the number of solutions or solution categories at pretest, indicating that the group selection process produced equivalent sets of subjects (Table 1). At posttest, however, the number of solutions and solution categories offered by trained children were both significantly greater than that of the control children ($p < .01$).

Behavior Rating Scale. The experimental group had significantly higher scores than the control group at pretest, but not at posttest. The teachers' ratings were determined to have been biased and therefore the data was disregarded.

Year 2

While the trained group was older than the control group, $\chi^2(1) = 17.37$, $p < .001$, analyses of all other demographics (sex, percentage attendance, sibling involvement, and family marital status) produced no significant differences between the groups. There was no behavior rating done this year because a reliable standardized rating scale had not yet been located.

Table 1

ANOVA OF Mean PIPS Subscale Scores

	Experimental		Control		
	Pretest	Posttest	Pretest	Posttest	Interaction Effect
			Year 1		
Solutions	5.5	6.2	4.9	3.1	5.58*
Categories	5.0	5.7	4.9	3.1	7.60**
			Year 2		
Solutions	3.6	7.1	3.3	4.7	6.67*
Categories	3.2	6.1	3.0	3.7	17.07**
			Year 3		
Solutions	4.4	8.4	4.2	4.5	14.78**
Categories	4.1	6.7	3.8	4.2	6.90*

Note. Year 1: n = 15 experimental, 14 control; Year 2: n = 15 experimental, 15 control; Year 3: n = 17 experimental, 18 control.

*$p<.05$. **$p<.01$.

PIPS. As with Year 1, a two-factor analysis of variance was used. The group means were similar on the number of solutions and the number of solution categories at pretest. Table 1 shows that from pretest to posttest there was a significant increase in the number of solutions ($p < .001$) and the number of categories of solutions ($p < .001$) for the experimental group only.

Year 3

On all but one of the outcome measures there were no differences between the two groups at pretest. The one significant difference, on the Hyperactivity/Distractable subscale of the PBQ ($t = 2.34$, $p < .05$), favored the control group.

PIPS. A two-factor analysis of variance was again used to assess the impact of interpersonal problem-solving training on cognitive ability and behavior. As indicated in Table 1, trained children showed a significant increase from pretest to posttest over their control counterparts on the number of solutions ($p < .001$) and solution categories ($p < .05$).

PBQ. Table 2 indicates that children who received training expressed fewer negative behaviors at posttest than did control children. Specifically, training had a significant moderating effect on children's anxious/fearful behaviors ($p < .001$), hyperactive/distractable behaviors ($p < .05$), and total negative behaviors ($p < .05$).

Other effects. The Headstart program had a contract with community mental health for consultation and service so that teachers could refer children about whom they had concerns. Trained children received significantly fewer referrals to the mental health consultant, $\chi^2(1) = 6.29, p < .05$, than did their control counterparts. This observed difference was consistent with the other treatment effects. It appears that training moderated the types of

Table 2

ANOVA of Mean PBQ Scores, Year 3

Condition	Hostility/ Aggression	Anxiety/ Fear	Hyperactivity/ Distractibility	Scale Total
Experimental (n = 17)				
Pretest	0.82	1.35	1.70	4.59
Posttest	1.00	0.24	0.88	2.76
Control (n = 18)				
Pretest	0.78	1.50	0.55	3.72
Posttest	1.11	2.89	1.11	5.78
Interaction effect	0.08	13.13**	5.23*	5.81*

*p<.05. **p<.001.

troublesome classroom behaviors that led teaching staff to seek outside professional consultation for a child.

Correlational analysis. The correlations presented in Table 3 between the pre-post change scores of the Solutions and Solution Categories subscales of the PIPS with the PBQ change scores provide support for the hypothesized link between cognitive skills and behavior. Not only were all correlations in the predicted direction, but also 38% of these correlations were found to be significant. The correlation between the direct measure of cognitive skill (Solutions) and classroom behavior (PBQ Total) was significant ($p < .05$). Thus, the pattern of these results suggest that changes in behavior which reflect better psychological adjustment are associated with improved ability to problem solve.

PIPS Change Scores

While three teachers provided training in the first year of the study, only one of those went on to provide the training in the second and third year. Therefore, the teacher who provided ICPS training in the second and third years had used the program before.

Table 4 shows the mean PIPS change scores across all three years. As expected, the PIPS change scores increased from Year 1 to Year 2 and to Year 3 for the number of Solutions and Solution Categories. This illustrates that as teachers become more experienced and comfortable with ICPS, their effectiveness will increase and greater improvement in the problem-solving abilities of children may be noticed in successive years of program implementation.

DISCUSSION

In all three years of the study, trained children showed a significant improvement in the number of Solutions and the number of Solution Categories over their control counterparts. This indicates that the trained children were better able to problem solve after training than were those who did not receive training.

The third year also found that trained children showed significantly fewer behavioral problems than did the control children. Significantly fewer referrals to the mental health consultant were made for the trained children than for the control children. Overall negative behavior and two of the three specific behaviors evaluated were significantly moderated for the children receiving training.

Table 3

Correlations Between Increase in Problem Solving Skills and Improvements in Behavior, Year 3 Experimentals

Preschool Behavioral Questionnaire Subscales	PIPS Scales	
	Solutions	Categories
Hostility/Aggression	.21	.17
Anxiety/Fear	.35*	.28
Hyperactivity/ Distractibility	.20	.22
Scale Total	.31	.30*

Note. *n* = 17.

*$p < .05$.

Table 4

Mean PIPS Subscale Pre-Post Change Scores for Trained Children

Year	PIPS Subscale	
	Solutions	Categories
Year 1 (*n* = 15)	0.7	0.7
Year 2 (*n* = 15)	3.5	2.9
Year 3 (*n* = 17)	4.1	2.6

Consistent with findings in previous studies for ICPS (Rickel & Burgio, 1982) and similar interventions (Weissberg, Cowen, Lotyczewski, & Gesten, 1983), however, aggressive behavior was not moderated by the training. The reinforcing nature of aggression is such that for antisocial children, disruptive behavior continues despite achievement of skills (Patterson, 1982).

The positive correlations found between the PIPS scales and the Preschool Behavioral Questionnaire corroborates Shure and Spivack's findings. The direct measure of cognitive skill (PIPS Solutions) was significantly and positively correlated with classroom behavior (PBQ total).

Thus, this Michigan replication of ICPS corroborates and adds further documentation to Shure and Spivack's findings. ICPS can be installed in an unsophisticated community setting with minimal investment of professional time. ICPS training improved problem-solving capability and classroom behavior in low-income rural preschool children. Further, behavioral changes which are reflective of psychological adjustment were associated with the improved ability to problem solve.

That these results were found with such small numbers suggests the strength of ICPS training when properly installed with dialoguing. The value of multiple year trials in community settings is suggested by the improvement of ICPS results with teacher experience. The continued evidence that aggressive behavior is less affected by interventions than anxious/fearful and hyperactive behavior argues for further developmental work. Nevertheless, the Newaygo study clearly established the value of ICPS as a preventive service model for community mental health.

REFERENCES

Behar, L., & Stringfield, S. (1974). A behavior rating scale for the preschool child. *Developmental Psychology, 10,* 601-610.

Cowen, E. L. (1977). Baby-steps toward primary prevention. *American Journal of Community Psychology, 5,* 1-22.

Gillespie, J. F., Durlak, J. A., & Sherman, D. (1982). Relationship between kindergarten children's interpersonal problem-solving skills and other indices of school adjustment: A cautionary note. *American Journal of Community Psychology, 10,* 149-153.

Patterson, G. R. (1982). *Coercive family process.* Eugene: Castalia Publishing Company.

Rickel, A. U., & Burgio, J.C. (1982). Assessing social competencies in lower income preschool children. *American Journal of Community Psychology, 10,* 635-645.

Ridley, C. A., & Vaughn, R. (1982). Interpersonal problem solving: An intervention program for preschool children. *Journal of Applied Developmental Psychology, 3,* 177-190.

Shure, M. B. (1976). *Staff training in a preventive mental health program* (Research and Evaluation Report #47, Consultation and Education Report #11). Philadelphia: Hahnemann Medical College and Hospital.

Shure, M. B. (1981). Social competency as a problem-solving skill. In J.D. Wine & M.D. Smye (Eds.), *Social competence* (pp. 158-185). New York: The Guilford Press.

Shure, M. B. (1982). Interpersonal problem solving: A cog in the wheel of social cognition. In C. Serafica (Ed.), *Social-cognitive development in context* (pp. 133-166). New York: The Guilford Press.

Shure, M. B., & Spivack, G. (1974/revised 1978). *A mental health program for kindergarten children: Training script.* Philadelphia: Department of Mental Health Science, Hahnemann Medical College.

Shure, M. B., & Spivack, G. (1979). Interpersonal cognitive problem solving and primary prevention: Programming for preschool and kindergarten children. *Journal of Clinical Child Psychology, 9,* 89-94.

Shure, M. B. & Spivack, G., (1980). Interpersonal problem solving as a mediation of behavioral adjustment in preschool and kindergarten children. *Journal of Applied Developmental Psychology, 1,* 29-44.

Shure, M. B., & Spivack, G. (1982). Interpersonal problem-solving in young children: A cognitive approach to prevention. *American Journal of Community Psychology, 10,* 341-356.

Spivack, G., Platt, J. J., & Shure, M. B. (1976). *The problemsolving approach to adjustment.* San Francisco: Jossey-Bass Publications.

Spivack, G., & Shure, M. B. (1974). *Social adjustment of young children: A cognitive approach to solving real-life problems.* San Francisco: Jossey-Bass Publications.

Weissberg, R. P., Cowen, E. L., Lotyczewski, B. S., & Gesten, E. L. (1983). The primary mental health project: Seven consecutive years of program outcome research. *Journal of Consulting and Clinical Psychology, 51,* 100-107.

Stress Management Training for Low-Income Women

Betty Tableman
Carolyn L. Feis
Michigan Department of Mental Health

Deborah Marciniak
Dennis Howard
Ionia County Community Mental Health Services Board

ABSTRACT. The stress management training model (SMT) was developed as a multi-dimensional program for low-income women. The program provided an introduction to life coping skills as well as a means of helping women feel better about themselves, take more control, accept responsibility, and learn about ways of handling stress. Two studies were conducted in Michigan: one as a prevention model and one as a treatment alternative. Findings from these two projects indicated that trained women were in better mood states and reported a greater perception of control than did women who did not receive such training. Services for SMT participants were also found to be nearly half as expensive as traditional one-on-one outpatient therapy.

One of the most successful of Michigan pilot demonstration projects has been a stress management training model (SMT) developed for women on public assistance in Ionia county, a rural area encompassing 577 square miles of central Michigan with a population of 50,000. The history of this project reflects often overlooked aspects of prevention programming: serendipitous confluence of professionals, technology, and community feasibility in determining what

---

SMT was developed initially by Diane Johnson, former prevention coordinator for Ionia County Community Mental Health, currently with the West Chester Counseling Center, Ohio, and by Roberta Rogers, Cooperative Extension Service. It was refined and documented by Deborah Marciniak. William L. Redmon and Pamela Luttig analyzed the data for the prevention project. Dennis Howard was responsible for the alternative treatment study.

Reprints may be obtained from Betty Tableman, Prevention and Demonstration Projects, Michigan Department of Mental Health, Lewis Cass Building, Lansing, MI 48926.

is done; the central importance of an effective recruiting process; the use of a psycho-educational approach; and the applicability of this technology for both prevention initiatives and alternative treatment.

SMT has run through the various steps of Michigan's model development and implementation process: demonstration and evaluation in Ionia county, documentation in a replication manual (Marciniak & Tableman, 1981), replication and evaluation in another site,[1] and dissemination. The evaluation of the model as an alternative treatment strategy, however, is unique to this project. This article will describe the development and content of SMT, the evaluation of the pilot demonstration prevention project, and the evaluation of SMT as an alternative treatment modality.

SMT was the unexpected outcome of an alliance between the community mental health center's prevention coordinator and a home economist from the cooperative extension service. Their mutual interest in stress management was first directed toward Type-A men at risk for physical consequences of stress. The target population was redefined in view of a needs assessment which showed low-income women with family problems to be substantial users of mental health services in Ionia county.

Women on public assistance characteristically exhibit low self-esteem and "learned helplessness" behavior as described by Seligman (1975). The economic realities of being on public assistance and the all too often destructive interpersonal relationships exacerbate stress and isolation for these women. Current difficulties and past traumas are seen as evidence of worthlessness; problems are perceived as unique and unmanageable. The combination of life stresses, low coping skills, and lack of a confiding relationship are strong precursors for depression (Brown & Harris, 1978).

SMT was developed as a multi-dimensional intervention to counteract these perceptions and behaviors. Cognitive restructuring was an essential first step to overcoming the women's perceptions of themselves as worthless and incapable of affecting their own lives. Theoretical work suggests that successful strategies to prevent or treat depression must modify attributions of worthlessness and expectations of failure (Hollon & Garber, 1980).

Behavioral training was also needed to enable these women to take control of their lives and to modify maladaptive responses. Low-income women characteristically use coping mechanisms that

[1] Analysis has not been completed on the replication of SMT in metropolitan Detroit.

exacerbate, rather than reduce, stress (Pearlin & Schooler, 1978). SMT incorporates a wide range of techniques and strategies, consistent with research suggesting that use of a variety of coping responses is more important in positive adjustment than any single specific response (Pearlin & Schooler, 1978; Spivack, Platt, & Shure, 1976). It was hypothesized that the impact of SMT would be shown in a reduction in the level of symptomatic feelings and moods and an increase in perceptions and attitudes indicative of control and competence.

The content of SMT was derived from mental health conceptualizations and research. Material from such diverse areas as stress management, social learning, values clarification, life planning, child abuse, and women's issues was translated into an intervention relevant for women on public assistance.

Other formulations related to learning contributed to the project design. SMT was a time-limited experience, using psychoeducational techniques. The group process provided support for change. Leaders participated as group members and shared their personal experiences, thus serving as role models. Learning was reinforced by "self-discovery" exercises done at home and a notebook to maintain handouts and exercises for future reference.

THE INTERVENTION

The Stress Management Training curriculum provided a broad introduction to life coping skills. It included: (a) cognitive restructuring toward a belief in one's power and potential; (b) techniques for life planning, i.e., setting and accomplishing goals and reducing life changes to manageable levels; (c) a framework for problem solving and decision making to change negative aspects of one's life; and (d) stress management skills and a repertoire of specific alternatives for reducing stress generated by unplanned or uncontrollable events.

The 10 week curriculum, as it was developed and used in Ionia county, was divided into three parts. The first three sessions were designed to enhance self-esteem and to identify stress-producing aspects of personal relationships (9 hours). The women explored the relationship between perceptions and self-esteem, began a process of self-discovery, and identified problems and goals on which to work. They learned to label feelings and to understand the difference between feelings and action. They explored the impact of negative feedback and practiced accepting and providing positive feedback. Also covered were steps toward developing a positive mental attitude, strategies for self-acceptance, attitudes toward women and women's roles, dynamics of destructive behavior, and positive approaches with children. Women explored communication and empathy in interpersonal relationships, how to meet needs, and how to respond to negative statements and actions. The concept of stress and relaxation through deep breathing was introduced in the third session.

The next five sessions on life planning (15 hours) covered acceptance of responsibility for behavior and techniques for taking control. Women clarified their values, needs, capabilities, and goals. They charted and let go of their past "Life Line" and projected a future "Life Line" (Kirn & Kirn, 1978). They explored decision-making approaches and practiced problem solving as well as making changes one step at a time. In addition, participants assessed key relationships in their lives, identified characteristics of "true" friends, and listed available personal and community supports.

Finally, in the last two sessions participants focused on understanding stress and stress management strategies (6 hours). They reviewed the signs of stress and the ways people respond to stressful situations. They learned stress-awareness and stress-resolution techniques. The women identified sources of personal stress and practiced anticipatory role playing, redefining the situation, and positive self-talk (Meichenbaum, 1975). They explored a range of positive coping strategies.

Groups ranged in size from 6 to 15 participants. Transportation and child care were provided to facilitate attendance. A snack break during the 2 1/2 to 3-hour sessions encouraged socialization and provided concrete opportunities to discuss nutrition. The intervention and service delivery are described in detail in the replication manual (Marciniak & Tableman, 1981).

STUDY 1: SMT AS A PREVENTION MODEL

Method

SMT was developed in Ionia county as a prevention model under funding from the Department of Mental Health. The pilot demonstration had an evaluation component to assess whether the intervention improved the capacity of low-income women to handle stress, as evidenced by proximal outcome indices of mental health status.

Participants

Participants in the Ionia county prevention project were white women with young children receiving Aid for Dependent Children (ADC), recruited by referral from the county Department of Social Services (DSS) and enrolled during a home visit. During the course of the evaluation, family service workers actively recruited women on their caseloads. The opportunity was offered to all women; participation was voluntary. When the family service positions were abolished, recruitment shifted to active pursuit of potential enrollees at the DSS office by a parttime person, a less effective procedure. Subsequently, with the initiation of the "workfare" program requiring participation of ADC recipients in education, training and job search activities, SMT became an option to which women with young children were routinely referred. During the period of the study, 65 women were enrolled as experimental subjects and 51 as controls. A random assignment procedure, alternating assignments upon receipt of names from DSS, was used.

Data was collected for 39 out of 45 women who attended at least 7 of the 10 stress management training sessions and 35 women who served as controls. The average age of participants was 28; the average educational level was 11th-grade, and more than three-fourths were one-parent families. There were no significant differences between experimental and control subjects on these characteristics.

Procedure

A pretest/posttest, nonequivalent control group design was implemented for the evaluation. Pretest data were collected in the month before the first workshop session. One posttest data collection point was selected, 3 1/2 months after the last workshop session (6 months after the pretest data) to ascertain whether SMT had any continuing effect. Participants were paid $3.00 for returning completed test data.

Measures

Measures selected were standardized instruments, comprehendible to low-income participants and relevant to the hypothesized impact of the training. In addition, a reporting form was developed by the project to capture satisfaction and impact of the training as perceived by the participants.

The Cornell Index. This 101-item checklist was designed to assess neuropsychiatric and psychosomatic symptoms (Weider, Wolff, Brodman, Mittelmann, & Wechsler, 1948). The total score and subscale score for Depression, Anxiety, and Inadequacy were used.

State-Trait Anxiety Inventory (STAI), Form X2. The measure of trait anxiety had 20 test items rated on a 4-point Likert scale in which the total score indicated how often a subject experienced various anxiety-related emotional states (Spielberger, 1968).

16 Personality Factor Test (16-PF), Form C. The 103 forced-choice item test measured 16 functionally independent, psychologically meaningful personality dimensions (The Institute for Personality and Ability Testing, 1969). Four dimensions were hypothesized as relevant to the training: Ego strength, Submissiveness/Dominance, Self-confidence, and Tension.

Consumer Evaluation A (Form A). This 20 item measure was developed specifically for SMT to assess participants' reactions to and satisfaction with the workshops. There were both open-ended and Likert-type items.

Results

Analysis of variance tests for pretest data on each outcome measure indicated significant pretest differences between experimental and control groups. A post hoc analysis of these effects showed the two groups differed significantly on six of nine factors, indicating nonequivalence prior to intervention.

This nonequivalence between groups required selection of an appropriate type of analysis as outlined by Cook and Campbell (1979): matching, analysis of covariance, or analysis of change scores. Matching was not feasible because of group pretest differences discovered after the fact. Analysis of covariance assumes that when pretest scores are regressed on posttest scores, the regression lines are comparable for experimental and control groups (Cohen & Cohen, 1975); the data did not support this assumption. An analysis of change scores was therefore used. Pretest scores were subtracted from posttest scores for each subject, and mean group change scores were compared for experimental and control groups using an independent-sample t-test.

Outcome Measures

Results in Table 1 show that experimental subjects improved significantly more than controls on Cornell Total and all three subscales, i.e., Depression, Anxiety, and Inadequacy, as well as on the STAI Trait-Anxiety scale and two of the four 16-PF subscales, i.e., Ego Strength and Self-confidence.

Table 1

Ionia County Prevention Project:

t-tests of Mean Pre-Post Change Scores

Measure Subscale	Experimental[a] (n = 39) Mean Change	 *SD*	Control (n = 35) Mean Change	 *SD*	*t*-test sign.
Cornell Index[b]	-8.74	12.80	0.06	7.53	< .001
Depression	-1.30	2.77	0.06	1.62	< .005
Fear, inadequacy	-1.74	3.93	0.00	1.92	< .005
Anxiety	-0.97	1.53	0.03	1.04	< .001
STAI -					
Trait-Anxiety[b]	-9.15	10.84	0.83	7.66	< .001
16 PF					
C-Ego strength[c]	1.79	2.44	0.09	2.37	< .001
E-Submissiveness/ dominance[c]	0.41	2.06	0.09	2.03	NS
O-Self confidence[b]	-1.69	3.02	0.43	2.29	< .001
Q -Tension[b]	-1.17	2.58	-0.74	2.19	< NS

[a] Completed 7-10 sessions.

[b] Negative change denotes better adjustment.

[c] Positive change denotes better adjustment.

Professional Observations

In addition to the evaluation measures, informal comments of professionals in contact with the women were noted. DSS staff indicated that ADC women who completed training, as compared to controls, made fewer "help me!" calls and, in times of crisis, were better able to participate immediately with the services worker in problem solving. Trained women, in comparison to controls, were described as more future oriented, talking about what they intended to do with their lives and when and how they would go about it. Women who had been uninvolved at Headstart meetings were reported to be actively participating and communicating their concerns. In other individuals, hostile and defensive behavior changed to more productive involvement.

Consumer Reports

Information about the perceived impact of training was collected from the women themselves. When posttest data was collected, women used the Consumer Evaluation to describe the value of the training and changes they had made in their lives as a result of participating in SMT. The following tabulation is based on comments made by 91 women who participated in SMT groups.

Women reported that SMT facilitated decision-making and change: 47% returned to school, obtained a job or a new place to live, resolved long-standing health problems, and made a decision to divorce or to accept this life change. One-third reported that they improved their relationships with children, husbands, boyfriends, and mothers while one-fourth reported that SMT resulted in better friendships, ability to use friends for support, and willingness to take time for themselves.

Thirty percent reported that they were more assertive in expressing their opinions and feelings, more in control of their lives, recognized that change was up to them, and were setting attainable goals. Thirty percent indicated that their outlook on life had improved; they felt more self-confident. Changes in cognition around problems and acquisition of problem-solving strategies were mentioned by 36%.

According to the women, the training sessions provided a rare opportunity for social contact, sharing, and acceptance ("I don't feel the world is against me anymore") and for recognizing that other people were also struggling. The workshops apparently helped the women to step back and look at their lives from a new perspective ("It made me think more about my life"), to talk over problems, and to find solutions in a way that they had never experienced before. Participants reported that they learned new concepts ("It's okay to look at the past and then let go of it," "To live one day at a time," "To plan for the future," "It's okay to make mistakes," "Take time for myself"). Training was said to change their expectations ("I am in control of my life; with time and effort I can change things") and their understanding of their own and others' needs. Training seemed to improve their ability to communicate and use their problem-solving skills ("I have a right to my opinion and feelings," "I got my husband to talk over problems instead of yelling and throwing things like I did before"). It reportedly enhanced assertiveness ("I'm not afraid to say no").

While these comments are anecdotal and limited to what the women selected to report, they do suggest how the women themselves perceived the impact of the training.

STUDY 2: SMT AS A TREATMENT ALTERNATIVE

Method

Although SMT was described in the replication manual as a prevention strategy, a survey of agencies who had purchased it indicated that several were using SMT in treatment settings. This suggested a broader relevance for SMT in community mental health services. To assess the impact of SMT, a psycho-educational group intervention, compared with traditional one-on-one outpatient therapy, a pilot was designed and evaluated in the Ionia county outpatient clinic.

Participants

Women from Ionia county who requested services from or were on the caseload of community mental health were randomly assigned by the staff evaluator to receive either SMT (n = 86) or traditional one-on-one outpatient therapy (n = 85). Women who were actively psychotic, severely depressed, or of borderline intelligence were excluded. Complete data was obtained for 59 women who received the training and 55 women who received outpatient therapy. Over half of the women who did not complete training responded to a questionnaire ($n = 17$). Eighty percent reported that scheduling conflicts, rather than the design or content of the workshops themselves, accounted for their lack of attendance.

Procedure

A pre/post equivalent group design was used. In order to understand better the pattern of change, it was decided to collect post-intervention data at two points in time. Pretest data was obtained at recruitment into the program, termination data at the end of training (10 weeks after enrollment), and follow-up data at 6 months after enrollment. The primary diagnoses of these women were equivalent across groups and consistent with the mental health center's outpatient caseload.

Women assigned to outpatient therapy were seen as frequently as they requested. Women assigned to SMT who were already on the caseload were also seen by outpatient therapists in accordance with their requests. Thus, the analyses do not provide for a comparison between SMT only and outpatient therapy.

Both groups were distributed equally across staff therapists. Staff therapists assigned to SMT and trained by the prevention coordinator were equivalent in training and experience to those delivering outpatient services.

Measures

In evaluating SMT as an alternative treatment, it was decided to retain the Cornell Index and the Consumer Evaluation for continuity with the previous study, to substitute two shorter measures for the lengthy 16-PF, and to add an easily administered, reliable measure for assessing mental health status.

Rosenberg Self-esteem Inventory. Nine Likert-type items, scored from 1 to 4, assessed the positiveness of one's attitudes toward oneself (Rosenberg, 1965).

Pearlin Mastery Scale. Seven items assessed the extent to which life changes were perceived to be within one's control or a result of fate (Pearlin & Schooler, 1978).

Progress Evaluation Scales (PES). Seven scales assessed current functioning (Ihilevich & Glaser, 1982) by five levels ranging from pathological to healthy. Assessed were: Family Interaction, Occupation, Getting Along With Others, Feelings and Mood, Use of Free Time, Problems, and Attitude Toward Self.

Results

Outcome Measures

Similar patterns of significant improvement ($p < .01$) were found for both groups on all measures except PES-Occupation from pretest to termination, and on all measures except PES-Family Interaction from pretest to follow-up (Feis, Tableman, Howard, & Marciniak, 1984). SMT women improved significantly more from pretest to termination than did the outpatient therapy participants (Table 2) on the Pearlin Mastery ($p < .01$) reflecting movement toward independence, and on the PES-Feelings and Moods subscale ($p < .05$). Through follow-up, this effect remained significant for both the measures ($p < .001$).

Consumer Reports

The suggestive information reported by SMT participants through the Consumer Evaluation was similar to that obtained from prevention workshop participants; however, percentages were lower.

Use of Outpatient Services

During the 10 week period of the workshop, 32 out of 59 SMT participants used outpatient visits. SMT participants averaged 2.39 outpatient visits (ranging from 0 to 19) plus 6.35 SMT sessions, while the outpatient participants averaged 3.71 visits (ranging from 0 to 43).

During the 14 week period between posttest and follow-up, 23 out of 59 SMT participants used outpatient visits, an overall average of 5.02 (ranging from 0 to 60); outpatient participants averaged 10. 98 visits (ranging from 0 to 169). Thus the mean number of outpatient therapy visits by SMT participants did not quite double while visits nearly tripled for outpatient participants during the period between posttest and follow-up. The maximum number of outpatient visits during the workshop for any SMT participant was less than half that for the highest outpatient-only participant; during the follow-up period, this number triples for SMT, but it quadruples for the outpatient group.

Cost Effectiveness

A cost analysis (including costs of outpatient visits made by SMT participants) was conducted at the 10 week termination and at the 6 month follow-up. The outpatient therapy cost was calculated as the number of visits × the length of visits × the agency cost per therapy

Table 2

Ionia County Treatment Alternative:

Test of Main Effects

Condition	Pretest	Termination Posttest	Pretest to Termination F^a	Followup Posttest	Followup F^a
			Pearlin Mastery		
SMT	9.31	6.59		6.90	
			15.22**		15.60**
Outpatient	8.61	8.84		8.55	
Interaction F^a			17.91**		11.85**
			PES-Feelings and Moods		
SMT	3.32	4.15		4.07	
			21.19***		11.69***
Outpatient	3.69	3.95		3.78	
Interaction F^a			6.31*		6.78***

Note. Low score represents greater mastery; high score represents more positive feelings and moods.

[a] $df = 1, 112$.

*$p<.05$. **$p<.01$. ***$p<.001$.

hour, divided by the number of participants. The costs for SMT was computed as 2 1/2 hours × 10 sessions × two persons × the agency cost per therapy hour, divided by the number of participants, plus the outpatient costs for these participants.

At termination, services used by the SMT were cheaper, with a mean cost of $143.11 per participant versus $150.84 mean cost per outpatient therapy participant. By the 6-month follow-up, the mean cost for outpatient therapy participants nearly tripled, averaging $446.42 while the mean costs for SMT participants did not even double, averaging $250.04. For the 6 month period, outpatient therapy cost nearly $200 more per client than SMT, while at the same time producing less effective results.

DISCUSSION

The history of SMT's development by field staff illustrates the translation of generative research into a prevention modality (Cowen, 1980). That SMT is also relevant as a treatment modality is not surprising: much of the generative research was developed in treatment settings. It underscores, however, that the major discriminator between prevention and treatment enterprises is not the characteristics of the intervention, but the point in time at which populations are accessed.

SMT was not unique in employing cognitive restructuring and behavioral training in a structured group format to prevent or modify maladaptive responses to stress and life change. Other such evaluated efforts (cf., Lewinsohn, Antonuccio, Steinmetz, & Teri, 1984; Roskin, 1982), however, have been directed at higher socioeconomic levels. SMT provided a format for exposing low-income women to elements of group support consciousness-raising, cognitive restructuring, problem-solving training, and other social competency and stress reduction techniques.

The data from the two Ionia studies suggest the strength of this approach. Changes in the women's perceptions and attitudes were reflected in the improvement in self-confidence and ego strength (16-PF) in Study 1 and the improvement in mastery (Pearlin), self-esteem (Rosenberg), and attitudes toward self (PES) in Study 2. Reductions in symptomatology were indicated in the Cornell Index (Study 1) and scores for feelings and moods and problems (Study 2). The comparison in Study 2 to traditional psychotherapy underscored the effectiveness of the psychoeducational approach.

These two studies, however, cannot tell us whether the results are a consequence of (a) the cognitive restructuring components, (b) the skill-building components modifying maladaptive behavior through facilitating life planning and problem-solving to change the negative aspects of one's life, (c) the repertoire of stress reduction strategies, or (d) the mobilization of social support. While a study to ascertain the one most effective component would be relevant, there is ample evidence that multiple pathways lead to and away from depression (Hollon & Garber, 1980; Akiskal & McKinney, 1973; Lewinsohn & Hoberman, 1982).

It has been suggested (Zeiss, Lewinsohn, & Munoz, 1979) that the critical components in a successful short-term cognitive-behavioral intervention included an elaborated well-planned rationale that guides the participant into the belief that she can control her own behavior, training in skills towards effectiveness in handling daily life, and encouragement of the participant's sense of mastery, i.e., that the participant not the professional is responsible for any improvement. These elements appear to be present in SMT.

The Ionia studies do not shed light on whether the changes evidenced are sustained over time beyond the 6 month period of the study. Specifically, Study 1 does not give us distal outcomes, i.e., whether SMT prevents depressive episodes and avoids use of mental health services for low-income participants confronted over time with increasingly harsh and capricious economic realities. It may well be that the significance of SMT is that by emphasizing control over one's response to events, modifying self-attributions, and increasing the coping repertoire, it positions participants when confronted with stress to use social support, to take advantage of formal assistance, and thus to restabilize more rapidly.

REFERENCES

Akiskal, H.S., & McKinney, W.T., Jr. (1973). Depressive disorders: Toward a unified hypothesis. *Science, 182,* 20-29.

Brown, G., & Harris, T. (1978). *Social origins of depression: A study of psychiatric disorder in women.* New York: Free Press.

Cohen, J., & Cohen, P. (1975). *Applied multiple regression/correlation analysis for the behavioral sciences.* New York: Wiley.

Cook, T.D., & Campbell, D.T. (1979). *Quasi-experimentation: Design and analysis for field settings.* Chicago: Rand-McNally.

Cowen, E.L. (1980). The wooing of primary prevention. *American Journal of Community Psychology, 8,* 258-284.

Feis, C.L., Tableman, B., Howard, D., & Marciniak, D. (1984). *Stress management training as an alternative treatment.* Lansing, MI: Michigan Department of Mental Health.

Hollon, S.D., & Garber, J. (1980). A cognitive-expectancy theory of therapy for helplessness and depression. In J. Garber & M. Seligman (Eds.), *Human helplessness: Theory and applications* (pp. 173-195). New York: Academic Press.

Ihilevich, D., & Glaser, G.C. (1982). *Evaluating mental health programs: The Progress Evaluation Scales.* Lexington, MA: Lexington Books.

Institute for Personality and Ability Testing (1969). *16 Personality Factor Test, Form C.* Champaign: Author.

Kirn, A., & Kirn, M.O. (1978). *Life work planning.* New York: McGraw-Hill.

Lewinsohn, P.M., Antonuccio, D.O., Steinmetz, J.L., & Teri, L. (1984). *The coping with depression course.* Eugene: Castalia Publishing Company.

Lewinsohn, P.M., & Hoberman, H. (1982). Behavioral and cognitive approaches to treatment. In E.S. Paykel (Ed.), *Handbook of affective disorders.* Edinburgh: Churchill-Livingston.

Marciniak, D., & Tableman, B. (1981). *Stress management training for women on public assistance: A replication manual.* Lansing, MI: Michigan Department of Mental Health.

Meichenbaum, D. (1975). A self-instructional approach to stress management: A proposal for stress inoculation training. In C.D. Spielberger & I.G. Sarason (Eds.), *Stress and anxiety* (Vol. 1.). New York: Wiley.

Pearlin, L.A., & Schooler, C. (1978). The structure of coping. *Journal of Health and Social Behavior, 19,* 2-21.

Rosenberg, M. (1965). *Society and the adolescent self-image.* Princeton: Princeton University Press.

Roskin, M. (1982). Coping with life changes: A preventive social work approach. *American Journal of Community Psychology, 10,* 331-340.

Seligman, M. (1975). *Helplessness: On depression, development and death.* San Francisco: W.H. Freeman.

Spielberger, C.D. (1968). *Self-evaluation Questionnaire: STAI X2.* Palo Alto, CA: Consulting Psychologists Press.

Spivack, G., Platt, J.J., & Shure, M.B. (1976). *The problem-solving approach to adjustment. A guide to research and intervention.* San Francisco: Jossey Bass.

Weider, A., Wolff, H.G., Brodman, K., Mittelmann, B., & Wechsler, D. (1948). *Cornell Index.* New York: The Psychological Corporation.

Zeiss, A.M., Lewinsohn, P.M., & Munoz, R.F. (1979). Nonspecific improvement effects in depression using interpersonal, cognitive and pleasant events focused treatments. *Journal of Counseling and Clinical Psychology, 47,* 427-439.

A Community Model for Prevention Services

Betty Tableman
Michigan Department of Mental Health

Deborah Marciniak
Ionia County Community Mental Health Services

Sue Bissell
Newaygo County Community Mental Health Services

ABSTRACT. Experience in Ionia county and Newaygo county in developing prevention services is described. These efforts, starting with needs assessment, illuminate principles underlying a community model for prevention services.

The Michigan program started out with an investigation of the prevention literature and a review of prevention programming as it then existed in a limited number of community mental health settings. There were a few ongoing prevention services: a social-emotional learning component in the schools, an ecological neighborhood intervention, parent training, and a preschool program for low income children. Beyond this, prevention programming was synonymous with consultation and education. To an outsider, these activities generally appeared to be episodic, without continuity or staying power. The percentage of time spent in developing materials seemed disproportionate to the time spent in service delivery. Programming seemed more responsive to the public relations and often casefinding needs of the agency and to the staff's interest in new challenges than to any systematic articulation of initiatives which might reduce the mental health agency's caseload.

The Ionia county program has had two prevention coordinators: Diane Johnson, 1976-1979, and Deborah Marciniak, 1979-present. The Newaygo county program has had three prevention coordinators: Charlotte Ellis, 1976-1978, Craig Simon, 1978-83, and Sue Bissell, 1983-present.

Reprints can be obtained from Betty Tableman, Michigan Department of Mental Health, Lewis Cass Building, Lansing, MI 48926.

The Michigan program set out to develop prevention service models to be installed as ongoing services in community mental health agencies. Characteristically, this has been undertaken by funding pilot demonstration projects which selected a specific target population and an intervention and proceeded to develop a defined prevention service. Two of the early projects, however, departed from this pattern: initially they were funded to explore appropriate parameters for prevention programming before settling down to a specific prevention initiative. While both projects did develop a specific prevention service, there also emerged from this initially unstructured venture a generalist approach to prevention programming—experience which could be translated into a community model for prevention services. This article will comment on what was learned in these two projects in terms of principles for a community model.

NEEDS ASSESSMENT

The projects were located in two western Michigan counties, Ionia and Newaygo, populations 50,000 and 35,000 respectively, adjacent to small metropolitan areas. Both counties undertook a needs assessment as the first step toward service development. The needs assessment included a review of the characteristics of the mental health center's caseload; an analysis of demographics and casualty data; and a review of the geography, ecology, and power structure of the area. Interviews with key informants verified risk populations and identified existing services and gaps in service.

It was anticipated that the needs assessment would structure subsequent programming. The needs assessment did turn up the general run of risk populations and a few unique risk situations. In Ionia county, for example, promising prevention targets were identified in the prison guards and their families who were high users of mental health services, the families of prisoners who migrated into the county, and a school system which annually extruded adolescents to the state hospital. Programming directed toward these specific situations, however, failed to develop, primarily because no community support or point of access emerged from the needs assessment process. The needs assessment made its major contribution in acquainting the prevention coordinator with the characteristics of the area and the cadre of professionals.

The survey of outpatient case files in Ionia county did indicate several suggestive trends. A high proportion of mental health center clients at that time were immature young adults, poorly prepared for the realities of adulthood, marriage, and childrearing. Anxious and depressed nonworking mothers of young children sought services around family conflict and childbearing. Many persons seeking treatment had been abused or neglected as children.

While the prevention coordinator identified stress management and the need for healthy parent-child relationships as relevant prevention themes, the core service actually evolved out of a relationship with a willing collaborator, a home economist on the staff of the Cooperative Extension Service, who shared the prevention coordinator's interest in the emerging stress management technology. Their initial efforts directed this "solution in search of a problem" toward men exhibiting Type A behavior. The reluctance of men's groups to participate in training and the results of the caseload analysis redirected the stress management training venture toward women on public assistance (see Tableman, Feis, Marciniak, & Howard, this issue).

In Newaygo county also, the needs assessment provided an introduction to the area and its professionals but did not clearly articulate a direction for development. The core service grew out of the availability of the Shure interpersonal cognitive problem-solving model and access to the Headstart program provided by a preexisting contractual arrangement with community mental health (see Feis & Simons, this issue). Subsequently a pilot demonstration on social-emotional learning was installed in the schools, growing out of a request for collaboration from the substance abuse agency. Thus, Newaygo county programming was initially directed at improving the coping capability of children.

Principle 1 then, in the emergence of a community service model, was that *the development of services related less to an assessment of "needs" than to the formation of community alliances, the testing of community interest, and the identification of feasible methodologies.*

CORE PROJECT: RECRUITMENT AND DISSEMINATION

If Phase 1 of these projects was the needs assessment, Phase 2 was the development and evaluation of the core service. The details of service delivery and evaluation are outlined in the articles referred to above.

Principle 2, in the formulation of the community service model, relates to all prevention service components developed under the Michigan program and is not unique to the community service model. That is, *recruitment of participants is undertaken via another service setting through which the population of concern can be systematically accessed.* Michigan prevention projects try to avoid the self-selection bias and haphazard process of open recruitment by forging collaborative linkages, e.g., systematic review of parents of newborns in the hospital setting (see Tableman & Katzenmeyer, this issue), referrals of divorcing or conduct-disordered families by courts, and linkages with mental health services to identify children of clients.

Both of the core projects exemplify this principle. Newaygo utilized the Headstart preschool setting for access to high-risk children and Ionia utilized various techniques through the county Department of Social Services (DSS), the most successful being recruitment by family services workers, when they existed, and subsequently routine assignment by employment and training staff. Other basic principles emerged after the development and successful evaluation of the core service, in Phase 3 of the Ionia project.

While prevention staff were interested in moving on to new challenges, the objective of the Michigan program was to pilot, evaluate, and install effective services models. The investment and thought going into model development was justified only if there was going to be sufficient exposure and penetration over time to make a difference. The state guidelines for continuation and transfer provided the mechanism for continued funding.

Accordingly, when the evaluation phase for the stress management training model was completed, the prevention coordinator continued to deliver stress management training (SMT) to women on public assistance, consistently running two to three concurrent groups. Then she began to branch out, still running the workshops herself but reaching somewhat different populations.

As an experiment under contract with DSS, she tried SMT with men on general assistance enrolled at the adult skills training center. She also used SMT with CETA trainees as part of a word processing training program and with a small group of rehabilitation clients.

The success of these efforts—the interest expressed in SMT by board members and others, and the indication from agencies from other areas that SMT was relevant to a broad range of populations—led to the next step: dissemination by spinning off responsibility for service delivery to other agencies. The determination was made by the mental health board and county director that the prevention coordinator should "saturate the community with stress management."

At various times, human service workers, adult education teachers, and student interns had been trained as co-leaders, learning the model by functioning as participant observers during regular workshop sessions. While this experience indicated that training facilitators was a feasible undertaking, there had been no consistent effort to give away SMT to other service systems.

The first such effort occurred in connection with the training of men on general assistance. Certified adult education teachers at the skills training center who had participated as co-leaders decided all of their students should be exposed to SMT; with consultation from the prevention coordinator, they implemented a mandatory class based on the SMT model but stressing employability issues.

A more comprehensive strategy for spinning off SMT to reach a broader population emerged in 1982 when a local community education director requested the prevention coordinator to teach a parenting course. The prevention coordinator offered to teach all of the community education teachers in the county to run the classes themselves; she suggested beginning with stress management rather than parenting, as self-awareness and effective coping skills are important basics for healthy parenting.

The community education directors accepted the proposal for stress management training-for-trainers and identified teachers who were certified, dependable, experienced, and good with people. Training included exposure to the model, active listening and group skills, and desensitization to sensitive topics (e.g., divorce, child abuse, incest, rape, alcoholism) that are inevitably raised during workshop sessions. The following year, parenting training-for-trainers was provided on a similar basis. SMT was installed as an adult education offering in four of Ionia county's five school districts.

In 1984, the prevention coordinator gave away a portion of SMT for women on public assistance to the special schools established as part of the employment and training program for welfare recipients. Community education teachers are now teaching stress management and life coping skills to women with children over six months of age who are enrolled in the program for high school completion.

These experiences suggested Principles 3, 4, and 5 of the community model of services: (3) *a core service will be developed,* (4) *this service component will be implemented with sufficient exposure and penetration over time to make an impact,* and (5) *where feasible, responsibility for service delivery will be delegated to other systems.*

LINKAGES AND COLLABORATION

As illustrated in the previous account, the prevention coordinator's work plan for SMT required collaborative linkages with social services, cooperative extension, and adult education staff. These relationships and others, in many ways, were a serendipitous outcome of the needs assessment process. In order to gain access to local informants, the prevention coordinator joined several coalitions focused on human services, prevention of child abuse, and employment services. She chose active participation in a few key organizations rather than passive involvement in a wider range of groups. These selected affiliations not only provided initial access to key informants; but more importantly, they laid groundwork for liaisons with professional colleagues and community agencies.

At the state level, there was no assumption that the prevention coordinator would go beyond the core service. At the local level, however, the prevention coordinator could not function as a specialist. The exploration and community linkages initiated during the needs assessment phase generated demands and expectations.

The coalition relationships provided linkages, organizational support, and community visibility for the prevention coordinator which would lead to various collaborative undertakings. Taking an active role in community groups led to leadership positions for the prevention coordinator because she was seen as committed and hardworking. As a result, she was able to get these groups to adopt, legitimize, and implement mental health priorities for prevention. The prevention coordinator also found that doing presentations consistent with her concerns before civic and church groups, high school classes, employees, etc., paid off in terms of visibility, credibility, and access to high-risk populations.

Principle 6 reflects this experience: *prevention services must develop linkages with other professionals as a base for service development; involvement with existing community coalitions are a means to this end.*

In Newaygo county, comparable opportunities for professional linkages did not exist, or were not used. Newaygo county developed an alternative approach for developing community input and support: an advisory committee which will be discussed in the next section.

Service Activities

Initial development of services in Ionia county represented an expanding partnership between the Department of Social Services and the prevention coordinator. More recent activities have involved other county agencies.

In addition to SMT, previously described, the prevention coordinator has worked collaboratively to support and upgrade parenting, to prevent teen pregnancy, to facilitate adjustment to divorce and to unemployment, and to promote health in the workplace. Two parallel and related themes link these efforts: enhancing the coping capability of adults and improving parenting. Similarly, two main modalities have been used: psycho-educational time-limited training and use of trained peers. These activities, undertaken in addition to the core service, are described below.

Parent aide program (1977-present). With funding for a staff position from VISTA, Prevention Services organized and ran a volunteer parent aide program for high risk and protective services families. For a time, DSS took over the volunteer recruiting and coordinating function, but staff cutbacks pushed this back to Prevention Services.

Unemployment response (1979-1981). In 1979, Chrysler announced that it was closing its Lyons Trim Plant, laying off almost 900 workers, primarily women. The state office suggested that the prevention coordinator become involved, in view of the research on unemployment and mental health. The prevention coordinator played a key role in organizing a community response intended to ease the transition and reduce disruptive effects for the unemployed individuals and their families. The prevention coordinator and the DSS director joined forces to found and co-chair the Chrysler Lyons Community Services Council. Council members represented the union, human services agencies, the business community, adult education, the employment security commission and other placement agencies, and local and state governmental units. Together they planned a proactive, collaborative response to the plant shutdown.

A peer counseling project was the most important Council activity. The Council decided that the peer counselors could be useful to the laid-off employees who were unable to accept that their jobs were really gone and reluctant to seek help at human service agencies. Three women who were community services representatives for the union were trained by the prevention coordinator to listen to their co-workers; scotch rumors about the plant closing; track down answers to questions about pensions, unemployment, and health insurance; make referrals to appropriate community resources; and advocate on behalf of co-workers who were struggling with bureaucratic organizations.

In addition, the Council served as a clearinghouse for persons wishing to return to school, ran workshops on stress and unemployment for agency staff who would be dealing with newly unemployed persons, and provided a forum for interagency communication and opportunities for peer counselors to air questions and concerns. The Council also sponsored group training sessions for the workers on everything from credit counseling to stress management, produced quarterly newsletters and compiled and distributed a community services directory.

Mobilizing the entire human services community to act together to respond to a catastrophe such as a plant closing offers endless possibilities for conflict around turf issues, broken promises, and personality clashes. While the Community Services Council was not altogether free from such problems, they were minimized by the previously formed relationships and trust among key actors.

Parenting course (1980). In response to interest expressed by DSS Protective Services, the prevention coordinator asked the youth service bureau and an Ionia community education teacher to collaborate on the development of a 16 session course on practical parenting skills. The course is offered by community education for high school credit. Scholarships for low-income persons who completed high school were provided by the local community services administration, and the child abuse prevention council provided money for transportation. This effort ultimately led to the expansion of SMT previously described.

Adolescent pregnancy (1983-present). The prevention coordinator became interested in adolescent pregnancy as an outgrowth of SMT, most participants having been adolescent mothers. As vice-chair of the child abuse prevention council, she persuaded the council to adopt adolescent pregnancy prevention as a priority and as a topic for the annual conference. When state project funding was made available for adolescent pregnancy prevention programs, the prevention coordinator wrote a grant proposal, underscoring the coalition sponsorship. A staff position, to be supervised by the prevention coordinator, has been funded to develop a parents newsletter and run workshops for middle and high school students and their parents.

Divorce (1984-present). The prevention coordinator is working with a circuit court family counselor to develop an orientation for divorcing parents to provide basic information on divorce and child custody issues and on available resources.

At the request of the Portland Area Ministerial Association, the prevention coordinator is also documenting a divorce adjustment group model she developed for a community education course. She will train lay persons affiliated with the ministerial association to reach out to the divorced in their community who need support during the period of adjustment.

Health promotion (1984-present). The prevention coordinator is working with the county health department and the personnel committee of the board of county commissioners to develop worksite health promotion, including stress management, for county employees. If successful, the program will be offered to the community at large.

Generalist Model

In these endeavors, the prevention coordinator sometimes initiated the effort and sometimes responded to interest or requests. The prevention coordinator has provided a capacity to organize, to access the literature, to develop grant proposals, and to train. Over time, the prevention coordinator has shifted away from direct service to facilitating service development, i.e., developing the component and then "giving it away" to the collaborating organization(s) (Principle 5).

This experience may be summarized in Principle 7: *the prevention coordinator in the community model functions as a generalist, moving to facilitate related facets of prevention programming beyond the core service as circumstances and community interest permit.* Abililty to accomplish this depends on the prevention coordinator using various mechanisms to expand her limited capacity (e.g., grant writing for additional funding and a training-of-trainers model).

ADVISORY COMMITTEE

In Ionia county, input for service development grew out of the affiliations with community coalitions. A more formal mechanism was adopted in Newaygo county as part of the effort to be accredited by the Joint Commission on Accreditation of Hospitals. JCAH standards for citizen input and participation provided the impetus for the organization of a prevention advisory council in 1980. The 13 members appointed by the mental health board for 3-year terms have variously represented the schools, clergy, social services, courts, public health, law enforcement, commission on aging, substance abuse agency, local newspaper, industry, and interested citizens.

Quarterly meetings provide the opportunity for members to review prevention activities and to address community needs. The advisory council has been responsible for encouraging the facilitation of the American Cancer Society's "I Can Cope" training for cancer patients and their families, undertaken by a community member (1980-present); the development of an annual interagency senior citizen's day (1982-present); accomplishment of two workshops for the unemployed (1982), and a parenting workshop for low functioning parents (1983). In 1984 the prevention advisory council was incorporated as a subcommittee into a broader advisory council covering outpatient and domestic crises, as well as prevention services. The new advisory council has questioned the piecemeal approach to programming evidenced to date, and staff is currently engaged in formulating a prevention plan to guide future development.

In addition to its input on programming and priorities, the advisory council in Newaygo county provides a means for involving community leaders, thus consolidating community support for prevention programming. In Ionia county, this process has been similarly accomplished through the community coalitions and also through on-going reporting to the county mental health board. Concerns expressed by a board member ("I have always been suspicious of prevention") led to the county mental health director placing the prevention coordinator on the agenda routinely for a report on her activities.

Principle 8 for the community model of services proposes *an explicit mechanism which enables prevention staff to communicate prevention concerns to the board, directly or through an advisory council.*

STAFFING

In Ionia county, the prevention function was set up as a clearly identifiable discrete activity reporting to the director of the agency. Prevention Services has a full-time coordinator and clerical assistant as well as its own stationery, telephone, and location (the latter since 1983, a case of necessity, not planful decision). This separateness in many ways increases the isolation from the rest of the staff inherent in a community-focused assignment.

In Newaygo county, on the other hand, prevention staff was integrated into outpatient services so that staff time was not 100% allocated to prevention but "traded off" with outpatient staff. Observation of the two projects from the state level suggests that the latter arrangement is less effective because of the diversion of attention and energy. Principle 9, therefore, specifies *full-time staff with no assignments outside of prevention.*

The experience in these two projects illuminates the qualitative differences between prevention coordinators and mental health therapists. The prevention coordinator must be capable of using psycho-educational and other nontraditional interventions and must be creative in translating mental health principles. Clinical understanding must be balanced by community organization and consultation skills and the ability to work collaboratively, avoiding turf issues and sharing the credit for accomplishment.

Prevention coordinators can accomplish nothing without the backing of other agencies and constituent groups, and must therefore invest themselves wholeheartedly in community organizations. Outpatient therapists can isolate themselves from the rest of the human services community and still get their jobs done. They do not require the cooperation of the other human services providers because they view their work as something only they can do, off with their clients, behind closed doors. If outpatient therapists do join community coalitions for public relations or casefinding purposes, they can afford to be relatively passive members.

DISCUSSION

We have reviewed the evolution of prevention services in two counties, deriving from that experience some principles for a community model. The components of the community service model can be summarized as follows:

1. A full-time prevention coordinator who operates as a generalist.
2. A core prevention service which is sustained and extended over time.
3. Development of other services consistent with community interest, circumstances and feasible methodologies.
4. Development of linkages with other professionals, including participation in community coalitions for service planning and development activities.
5. Recruitment of service participants through systematic access.
6. Collaborative service arrangements and emphasis on approaches which will expand service capacity.
7. Spin-off of prevention services to other community agencies.
8. An advisory committee representative of the community and/or routine arrangements for reporting to the board.

There is another dimension that has not been discussed: the community model should have an explicit or implicit plan for the development of services.

Neither of the two projects described have had an explicit plan for prevention services. Nor is it clear that an explicit plan detailing all proposed moves is strategically wise.

The experience in these projects does suggest, however, that there should be some formulation related to the areas and populations of concern and to the conceptual and methodological approach to programming. Whether the mental health setting selects empowerment of adults, as in Ionia, or improving the interpersonal cognitive problem-solving skills of children, as initially in Newaygo, is less important than that there be a focus. Whatever the primary approach selected—time-limited psycho-educational training, behavior modification or interpersonal cognitive problem solving, self-help or trained peers—is less important than that the choice be made with knowledge of strengths and limitations, and a clear rationale.

In the absence of such a core formulation, the prevention program will be vulnerable to passing fancies and diversion of resources with no clear sense of direction or purpose. Developing and sustaining prevention services is a balancing act, putting together community needs, theoretical constructs and methodology from the literature, and collaborative linkages, all in the context of a constantly changing scene. Community crises arise, collaborators move on, funding sources wax and wane. It helps to have stable constructs around which efforts can continue to be organized.

Exploring Work as an Arena for Prevention Research: The Michigan Prevention Research Center

Richard H. Price
James House
Jeanne Gordus
University of Michigan

ABSTRACT. This article offers a rationale and reviews the research evidence for a focus on work transitions in prevention research. The organization and current research of the Michigan Prevention Research Center are then described. Current research and dissemination activities are presented in the context of a prevention research cycle that moves through four domains: problem analysis, intervention design, evaluation, and knowledge dissemination.

Evidence is accumulating indicating that a variety of work transitions are associated with increases in stress, maladaptive patterns of coping and enduring negative health and mental health outcomes in vulnerable populations (e.g., Catalano & Dooley, 1980; Gordus & McAlinden, 1984; House, 1981; Kahn, 1981; Price, 1984). Furthermore, a recent review has shown that a variety of forms of naturally occurring social support from family members, co-workers, supervisors and others can directly reduce work related stress and buffer its impact on these vulnerable populations (e.g., LaRocco, House, & French, 1980).

The impact of work transitions and strains may have particularly deleterious effects on vulnerable populations such as those with already diminished sources of support, the elderly, and minority

---

This paper was supported by Grant MH38330 from the Office of Prevention Research, National Institute of Mental Health to the Michigan Prevention Research Center. Reprints may be obtained from Richard H. Price, Director, MPRC, Institute for Social Research, Box 1248, University of Michigan, Ann Arbor, MI 48106.

groups, and may reach beyond the worker to family members and children (e.g., Liem & Rayman, 1982) as well. Correspondingly, these groups may benefit from effective preventive interventions designed to enhance coping capacity.

What is now needed are preventively oriented field experiments to test the effects of various forms of support on work related stress and enduring mental health and health outcomes. Experimental field trials provide the opportunity to develop preventively oriented programs based on successful field experiments that can be disseminated widely both in the workplace and in mental health and social service agencies (Price, Ketterer, Bader, & Monahan, 1980; Price 1982a,b). At the same time, work, a major life sphere, and the workplace itself represent a substantially neglected arena for the conduct of preventive research in mental health, and a major opportunity for prevention research (Price, 1984, in press).

Most social service agencies and community mental health centers have not played a major role in the development of preventively oriented programs to deal with work transitions in the past. The opportunity exists, we believe, to conduct survey research and field experiments that could form the basis for preventive programs in the future. In what follows we describe rationale and activities of the Michigan Prevention Research Center. The objectives of the Center are to (1) establish a multidisciplinary group of researchers who will conduct epidemiological oriented surveys and analyze existing survey data to explore the mental health and health impacts of job transitions, (2) conduct field experiments to test the effect of programs designed to prevent enduring negative health and mental health impacts on high risk populations, (3) disseminate program findings both in Michigan and nationally to mental health and other service providers and as well to researchers, and (4) to develop empirical and theoretical knowledge on the prevention of negative mental health and health consequences of work stress and work transitions.

CHANGES IN THE LABOR MARKET IN THE '80s AND BEYOND

A focus on work transitions such as unemployment and job changes within the worksite is not a short term response to current economic changes, but to long term changes anticipated in the labor market in Michigan and nationally. Both job shifts, loss of employment and career plateaus, all potentially highly stressful experiences, will become widespread. Future projections (Flaim & Fullerton, 1978) indicate that between 1982 and 1990-4, there will be severe and continuing job loss, downward employment mobility, and job shifts.

Employment grew in America throughout the 1970s at an annual average rate of 2.1 percent, an unprecedented high, compared with the 1960s average of 1.5 percent (Pursell, 1980). This growth served to accommodate in part, a substantial increase in the numbers of Americans seeking work. The baby boom generation began to enter the work force in 1963 and more rapidly in greater numbers thereafter until the late 1970s. Women began to participate in the labor force at a rapidly increasing rate. Finally a large number of returning Vietnam veterans attempted to enter the labor force, putting yet more pressure on employment opportunities. Despite employment growth, a shortage of jobs was felt among lower socioeconomic groups, particularly minorities, youth and women, and those lacking specialized job skills.

The best estimates indicate that substantial job loss and job change will continue to occur (Flaim & Fullerton, 1978; Pursell, 1980). The 1978 automotive labor force of 977,000 is expected to stabilize at 550,000 in 1985. Thus, a population which had a relatively high level of risk for unemployment, but which has had employment in the past, will have its employment opportunities constrict continually during the next decade or so. Few alternatives except highly stressful life changes—retraining, relocation and/or drastically reduced living standards and concomitantly changed family functioning—will be available to them (Ferman & Gordus, 1979).

IMPACT OF WORK TRANSITIONS

There is now a broad array of evidence available to suggest that employment transitions and unemployment, in particular, are associated with a variety of negative health and mental health outcomes (Gordus & McAlinden, 1984). The evidence included case studies of the unemployed and profiles of families of the unemployed collected during the depression (Zawadzki & Lazarsfeld, 1935) and more recently (Slote, 1969) indicating increases in depression and marital conflict. Still another set of studies relating aggregate economic conditions such as unemployment rates to aggregate indicators of social and psychological disorder (Brenner, 1976) has suggested that there are relationships between economic conditions and rates of mental hospital admissions, suicide rates, and rates of stress related illnesses. These aggregate level studies remain somewhat ambiguous with respect to the causal relations between individual circumstances of unemployment and individual psychological outcomes (Kasl, 1979).

However, recently Catalano and Dooley (1980) have reviewed the evidence for the relationship between economic life change and subsequent outcomes. Their analysis of individual level longitudinal studies (Cobb & Kasl, 1977; Cohn, 1978; Parnes & King, 1977; Schlozman & Verba, 1979) suggests that there is considerable evidence that changes in employment status and unemployment, in particular, are associated with a variety of negative social and mental health outcomes. While the evidence that there is an association between employment status change and psychological distress continues to develop, the etiological mechanisms associated with changes in employment status remain to be specified. For example, Catalano and Dooley (1979) suggest that economic change may uncover some already existing behavioral disorders rather than play a role only as provoker of those disorders. It may be that both uncovering and provoking mechanisms operate and contribute to overall rates of psychological disorder.

Nevertheless, the evidence suggests that a very broad range of negative health and mental health outcomes are observed as a consequence of changes in employment status. These negative impacts are not uniformly observed in the population experiencing employment transitions or unemployment. For the purposes of developing effective preventive interventions, the question of what groups are specifically at highest risk for negative health and mental health outcomes is of considerable importance.

Social support as a protective factor. One important line of evidence concerning the question of who is at risk for psychological distress and disorder as a consequence of unemployment is offered by Kasl and Cobb (1979). These investigators studied male industrial workers in two plants over a two year period during which the plants were closed and the men lost their jobs of long-standing and had to seek new employment. The men were interviewed concerning occupational, financial, familial, and health status in anticipation of scheduled closing, at termination itself, and six months, twelve months, and twenty-four months after the plant closing. For our purposes, the salient finding obtained by Kasl and Cobb has to do with the relationship between psychological symptoms of depression and perceived social support. Those workers who perceived themselves as having relatively low levels of social support and who were unemployed for longer periods had systematically higher levels of symptoms of depression and work role deprivation than other groups who perceived themselves as having higher levels of social support. House (1981) interprets the Kasl and Cobb findings to suggest that the negative effects of unemployment on depression are largely eliminated by adequate social support and that these data suggest that social support has the potential to buffer the negative effects of stress on individuals experiencing unemployment.

The meaning of low perceived social support in the Kasl and Cobb (1979) study and numerous others is complex. Reports of lower levels of social support may reflect *both* differences in objective social conditions and a complex of attitudes and attributions towards both the self and social environment (Brickman, Rabinowitz, Karuza, Coates, Cohn, & Kidder, 1982; Bowman, 1982; Cohn, 1978). Nevertheless, it seems clear that persons holding different perceptions of the availability of support and their capacity to control the environment are at differential risk for negative psychological outcomes associated with employment transitions.

Stages of the unemployment experience. A second critical variable in determination of risk has to do with the phases of adaptation and adjustment to the experience of unemployment. Jahoda (1979), Kaufman (1982), and King (1982) all suggest that several distinctive stages in the pattern of adaptation to unemployment can be discerned. They include a stage of anticipation which begins when the possibility of job loss is perceived. The anticipatory phase often is characterized by denial and disbelief, anxiety reactions, and accompanying defensive responses. The second stage, actual job loss, is a stage in which the uncertainty of anticipation is resolved. This stage is characterized by a period of relaxation and relief and optimistic attitudes about the possibility of reemployment (Powell & Driscoll, 1973). Frequently, this second phase is also characterized by job search activity or increased receptivity to labor market search. If, however, the job search is ineffective, a third stage of adaptation to prolonged unemployment ensues with a proliferation of negative stress reactions and emergence of a variety of psychological symptomatology. This stage may be characterized by intense moodiness, anxiety, depression, feelings of panic, rage, self-doubt, social withdrawal, increased alcohol and drug abuse, marital disorganization, and other adverse psychological reactions.

In addition to these adverse psychological reactions, some researchers (Buss, Redburn, & Waldron 1983) suggest that increased social isolation may develop in this third stage. Thus, one's network of social support may be eroded in times of prolonged unemployment. This stage oriented formulation should be regarded as hypothesis rather than fact and subject to a variety of influences. If however, such a sequence of events marks the course of unemployment, then efforts to reduce the duration of unemployment should have preventive impacts.

While we have focused on the experience of unemployment in our discussion thus far, a variety of work transitions such as retirement, promotion, and job change as well as chronic work stresses, including jobs with high demand and low control or support, may also place workers at risk for negative health and mental health outcomes (House, 1981; Kahn, 1981; Price, 1984; Price & Bronfman, 1984). The Michigan Prevention Research Center, which is described in the remainder of this paper, has as its major goal the identification of risks and protective factors associated with work transitions, and the development and testing of preventive programs aimed at reducing those risks.

THE MICHIGAN PREVENTION RESEARCH CENTER

The Michigan Prevention Research Center (MPRC) has several key features: (1) MPRC focuses on one aspect of adult life—paid employment or the lack thereof—which in varying ways may play a major role in the development of health and mental health problems and provides organized channels for effective intervention to prevent the development of those disorders, even those whose etiology is wholly or partially non-work-related. (2) MPRC brings together, in programs of intervention and research, professionals with experience and skill in epidemiologically oriented survey research and persons with experience and skill in processes of intervention design, implementation and evaluation (cf., Price, 1982b). The Center has been funded by the Center for Prevention Research, National Institute of Mental Health, since September, 1983.

We see work and the work place in our proper focus for several reasons. First, as we suggested earlier, substantial evidence indicates that chronic psychosocial stress at work and/or major occupational transitions significantly increase the risk of psychological disorder among persons exposed to these stresses or transitions and their families (e.g., Brenner, 1973; Caplan, 1975; Ferman & Gordus, 1979; House, 1980; 1981; Kahn, 1981; Kornhauser, 1965).

Second, work organizations (including employers and unions or occupational associations) provide the effective channels for implementing intervention programs aimed at preventing mental/emotional disorder among adults. That is, work organizations are for adults what schools are for children—a social organization where they spend a major portion of their waking hours. They are not only a potent source of both stress and positive rewards, but also contain ready made channels for disseminating and implementing preventive mental and physical health programs. Thus, both because the work experience is significant for well being and because the worksite lends itself to prevention programming, MPRC is concerned with the preventive possibilities in the work arena.

The Michigan Prevention Research Center combines several streams of research activity and program development into a new program of prevention research on work related stress and coping. The program brings together several cooperating organizations into a programmatic effort that combines the research expertise of researchers at the Institute for Social Research and the Institute for Science and Technology at the University of Michigan with the mental health system in Michigan, particularly the Prevention and Demonstration Projects Unit at the Michigan Department of Mental Health and the Washtenaw County Community Mental Health Center.

Each of these organizations has its own history of work on prevention in mental health and/or job transitions and stress. Their collaboration in the context of MPRC produces a prevention research capacity of considerable scope and depth. In addition, the MPRC group is multidisciplinary in character, including psychologists, sociologists, public administrators, a labor market economist, and therefore brings a wide array of perspectives and skills to the organization. The current MPRC faculty is listed below.

—Richard H. Price, MPRC Director, Professor of Psychology, and Faculty Associate in Survey Research Center, Institute for Social Research, University of Michigan

—Saul Cooper, Director, Washtenaw County Community Mental Health Center and Adjunct Professor of Psychology, University of Michigan
—Jeanne P. Gordus, Associate Research Scientist and Lecturer, Institute for Science and Technology, University of Michigan
—James S. House, Program Director, Social Environment and Mental Health Program, Survey Research Center, Institute for Social Research and Professor of Sociology, University of Michigan
—Robert L. Kahn, Professor of Psychology and Research Scientist in Survey Research Center, Institute for Social Research, University of Michigan
—Ronald C. Kessler, Faculty Associate, Survey Research Center, Institute for Social Research and Associate Professor of Sociology, University of Michigan
—Ruth Fine Schelkun, Coordinator of Community Services, Washtenaw County Community Mental Health Center
—Betty Tableman, Director, Prevention and Demonstration Projects Unit, Michigan Department of Mental Health
—Paul Wortman, Professor in School of Public Health and Director, Methodology and Evaluation Research Program, Center for Research on Utilization of Scientific Knowledge, Institute for Social Research, University of Michigan

The Prevention Research Cycle

We conceptualize our research as moving through the prevention research cycle (Price, 1982a, 1984). A schematic description is shown in Figure 1 and guides our conceptualization of the prevention intervention research process. Briefly, it depicts a series of research cycles that we believe are necessary to move from an (1) initial problem analysis of the prevention research problem to (2) the design of a preventive intervention, (3) to the actual field testing and evaluation of the intervention, and finally to (4) the dissemination of the program to populations of individuals, groups or agencies that can provide wider preventive impact such as mental health centers, unions, and community agencies. While we recognize that these various cycles do not always occur in an entirely sequential fashion, the framework does provide a conceptual map to orient us in planning and implementing research activities and to measure progress toward prevention goals.

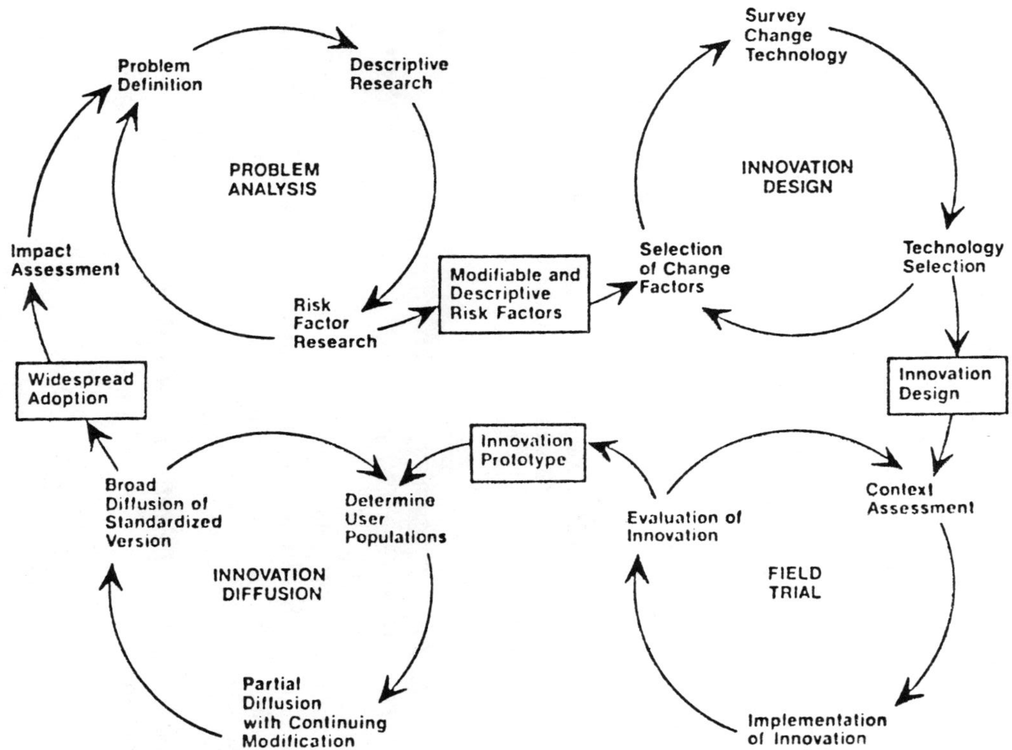

Figure 1. Four Domains of Prevention Research.

In addition, our research plan is designed to link broad based epidemiological survey research with our design of preventive intervention (Price, 1982b). Thus, results of our survey research activities can provide us with information concerning the nature and extent of problems and risk factors encountered by populations in the community experiencing various work transitions. Survey research in the workplace can also allow us to identify workers who do not yet anticipate a work transition, but who have a reasonably high likelihood of doing so in the near future. This orientation provides the opportunity to engage in "reactive" primary preventive intervention research aimed at helping displaced workers cope with the stresses of unemployment and their health and mental health sequelae and to engage in "proactive" prevention research designed to modify conditions in the workplace and worker capacity to cope with them before they occur (Catalano & Dooley, 1980). Thus, the range of research activities and research sites we plan to undertake will allow us to examine both stressful life events such as work transitions and worker dislocation on the one hand, and more chronic work stresses and role strains that characterize many work roles in organizational settings on the other.

CURRENT ACTIVITIES AND FUTURE PLANS OF THE MICHIGAN PREVENTION RESEARCH CENTER

In the remainder of this paper we will briefly describe some of the current research activities and future plans of MPRC. We will use the stages of the prevention research cycle as an organizing framework.

Problem Analysis: Identification of Risk Factors in Work Transitions

A primary objective of MPRC is to link epidemiologically oriented survey research findings to the design of preventive interventions. This is both a methodological and conceptual task that is critical to the accurate targeting and effective design of preventive interventions. Epidemiologically oriented survey data can inform the design of preventive interventions in several ways. First, epidemiological surveys can clarify questions about the extent and distribution of work related problems in the community and allow estimates of relative risk. Second, such information can aid decisions about the potential value of mounting a preventively oriented program. In addition, survey results can help to clarify some of the linkages between short term responses to unemployment or stressful work conditions and more enduring mental health and health outcomes. These points of linkage are potential targets for intervention once they are identified. Third, survey research can aid in the identification of variables that identify those groups at highest risk for psychological disorder and, therefore, provide better definitions of the target population for intervention programs. Finally, survey research can identify help-seeking patterns in the community and estimate utilization rates for various help sources. Such information is useful in building organizational linkages and referral networks between existing services and newly developed preventive programs.

During our first year, our survey team, led by sociologists James House and Ronald Kessler, has developed and field tested a survey instrument focused on unemployment and psychological well being. They are currently conducting interviews with a sample of employed and unemployed workers in the Washtenaw county area to assess the mental health impacts of unemployment. The sampling design of this survey allows us to interview (1) a probability sample of currently unemployed workers, as well as (2) a sample of employed workers who have experienced a period of unemployment in the past five years, and finally (3) a sample of employed workers who have not experienced such an interruption in employment. The survey asks each respondent about: social support, life events, personality dispositions, marital life, parental behavior, characteristics of the employment and unemployment experience, financial support, symptoms of mental disorder, patterns of help-seeking, and demographic characteristics.

A second wave of this survey will be conducted in approximately one year. This second wave will allow us to obtain important longitudinal data on these samples which will strengthen our capacity to make causal inferences about the impact of work transitions on health and mental health. In addition, we expect to sample a small subgroup during the second wave for much more intensive interviews. These intensive interviews should provide more detailed mental health assessments that are not possible in most community surveys. We anticipate that this series of epidemiologically oriented surveys will substantially increase our knowledge about the role of work transitions and associated life events in the development of health and mental health disorders.

A second research project focused on the mental health and health impacts of job transitions is directed by evaluation researcher Paul Wortman, one of our MPRC faculty, in collaboration with organizational psychologist Robert Kahn and Richard Price. This project will examine existing research literature on occupational stress and conduct a number of systematic analyses of the impact of work stressors on alcohol, mental health and drug abuse outcomes. The method of analysis in this project will be data synthesis (Wortman, 1983; Yeaton & Wortman, in press). Data synthesis is a method for quantitative synthesis of data from diverse studies in order to obtain more reliable estimates of the effect of variables of interest.

We expect that this systematic examination of research findings in this field will lead to information about potential risk factors associated with occupational stress. We see these two risk factor research projects as complementary in their focus and expect they will increase our understanding and knowledge of risk factors associated with work transitions.

Intervention Design and Evalution

Our Center is also designing and evaluating intervention programs intended to prevent enduring negative health and mental health impacts of work transitions. Our current work is focused on the evaluation of the Employment Transition Program developed by labor market researcher Jeanne Gordus. The ETP is a five day group oriented program oriented to education, cognitive restructuring, and behavioral skill acquisition (Catalano & Dooley, 1980) for persons experiencing unemployment and job transitions. Specifically, ETP is designed to (1) help workers identify and use personal, familial and interpersonal resources, (2) increase information about the labor market, (3) increase knowledge about employer behavior and job search strategies and, (4) to improve job search skills. The preventive rationale underlying ETP is that reducing the duration of the unemployment experience and enhancing skills to cope with the stresses of job search should reduce the likelihood of negative health and mental health outcomes.

During the past year, developmental work on recruitment, delivery, assessment, and evaluation of the Employment Transition Program was conducted. These pilot replications and the recruitment studies should allow an effective implementation and evaluation of the Employment Transition Program in the second year of our MPRC project. In addition, both formative and outcome evaluation instruments were designed to assess (1) delivery of the program, (2) knowledge acquisition of participants, (3) actual use of information from the program in coping, and (4) assessment of the health and mental health impact for experimental and control groups.

An additional affiliated research project directed by organizational psychologist Robert Caplan will begin in 1985 which will evaluate a different version of the Employment Transition Program to aid unemployed workers to re-enter the labor market. This study should substantially increase our capacity to understand the effect of systematically developed social support strategies (Janis, 1983) in coping with work transitions. These two field experiments will provide us with complementary information on distinctively different populations at risk for negative mental health outcomes associated with work transitions.

Finally, an affiliated research project, directed by public health researcher Barbara Israel in collaboration with organizational researcher Susan Schurman and sociologist James House, is being conducted to evaluate the effectiveness of an action research approach for the prevention of occupational stress-related alcohol, drug abuse and mental disorders. The project emphasizes a participative approach and will be conducted in a local automotive parts manufacturing plant.

Dissemination Activities

The Center has engaged in a variety of dissemination activities in the past year. First, under the direction of Jeanne Gordus, MPRC was a co-sponsor of the national conference on Coping with Unemployment. The conference was designed for union representatives, mental health agency personnel, employment and training professionals, and other interested practitioners in the field. The objectives of the conference were to integrate the best of mental health, labor, and other human service agency approaches to unemployment and to provide information to aid practitioners in serving the unemployed. The conference featured workshops on one-day assistance programs, unemployment centers, overcoming barriers to community responses, recruiting, and pre-layoff interventions. We anticipate that this activity will be repeated in future years in other states as part of our dissemination strategy.

MPRC staff have also been identifying promising intervention programs and developing descriptions of these programs. We hope to use these descriptions to create a clearinghouse which will provide information to practitioners throughout the field who wish to develop their own local programs. In a parallel effort, MPRC staff has developed an annotated bibliography of research literature on risk and protective factors in unemployment and occupational stress (Price & Bronfman, 1984). This and other research reports and program materials will be made available to interested researchers and practitioners in the field.

CONCLUSION

While our work in MPRC is still in its early stages, we have initiated a number of projects with complimentary goals at each stage of the prevention research cycle. As our exploration of various work transitions and stresses broadens, we anticipate an increasing focus on the workplace and the links between work and other life domains (Price, 1984, in press). A continuing theme of our research will be to strengthen the conceptual and methodological ties between survey oriented risk factor research on the one hand, and the development of interventions on the other. The testing of preventive interventions in field experiments allows us to design useful programs and to test scientific hypotheses about the causal status of risk factors at the same time. The experience of work, and the workplace itself, offers numerous challenges and opportunities for prevention. We are only now beginning to see the possibilities.

REFERENCES

Bowman, P. (August, 1982). Social psychology of discouragement among jobless black Americans: Research agenda, preliminary analysis, and implications. In P. Bowman (chair), *Problems of joblessness in black America.* Symposium presented at the meeting of the American Psychological Association, Washington, D.C.

Brenner, M.H. (1973). *Mental illness and the economy.* Cambridge, MA: Harvard University Press.

Brenner, M.H. (1976). *Estimating the social costs of national economic policy: Implications for mental and physical health, and criminal violence* (Report prepared for the Joint Economic Committee of Congress). Washington, D.C.: U.S. Government Printing Office.

Brickman, P., Rabinowitz, V., Karuza, J., Coates, D., Cohn, E., & Kidder, L. (1982). Models of helping and coping. *American Psychologist, 37,* 368-384.

Buss, T.F., Redburn, F.S., & Waldron, J. (1983). *Mass unemployment: Plant closings and community mental health.* Beverly Hills, CA: Sage Publications.

Caplan, N. (1975). *The use of social science knowledge in policy decisions at the national level.* Ann Arbor, MI: Institute for Social Research, The University of Michigan.

Catalano, R., & Dooley, D. (1979, December). Does economic change provoke or uncover behavior disorder? A preliminary test. In L. Ferman & J. Gordus (Eds.), *Mental health and the economy.* Kalamazoo, MI: W.E. Upjohn Institute for Employment Research.

Catalano, R. & Dooley, D. (1980). Economic change in primary prevention. In R.H. Price (Ed.), *Prevention in mental health.* Beverly Hills, CA: Sage Annual Review of Community Mental Health.

Cobb, S., & Kasl, S.V. (1977, June). *Termination: The consequences of job loss* (Report No. 76-1261). Cincinnati, OH: National Institute for Occupational Safety and Health, Behavioral and Motivational Factors Research.

Cohn, R.M. (1978). The effects of employment status change on self attitudes. *Social Psychology, 41,* 81-93.

Ferman, L., & Gordus, J. (Eds.). (1979). *Mental health and the economy.* Kalamazoo, MI: Upjohn Institute.

Flaim, P.O., & Fullerton, H.N. (1978). Labor market force projections to 1990: Three possible paths. *Monthly Labor Review, 101*(12), 25-36.

Gordus, J.P., & McAlinden, S. (1984, June 29). Economic change, mental illness, physical illness and social deviance. (Joint Committee of the U.S. Congress). Washington, D.C.: U.S. Government Printing Office.

House, J.S. (1980). *Occupational stress and the mental and physical health of factory workers.* Ann Arbor, MI: Institute for Social Research Report Series.

House, J.S. (1981). *Work stress and social support.* Reading, MA: Addison-Wesley.

Jahoda, M. (1979, August). The impact of unemployment in the 1930's and the 1970's. *Bulletin of the British Psychological Society, 32,* 309-314.

Janis, I.L. (1983, February). The role of social support in adherence to stressful decisions. *American Psychologist, 38,* 143-160.

Kahn, R.L. (1981). *Work and Health.* NY: Wiley.

Kasl, S. (1979). Changes in mental health status associated with job loss and retirement. In J. Barrett (Ed.), *Stress and mental disorder.* New York: Raven Press.

Kasl, S., & Cobb, S. (1979). Some mental health consequences of plant closing and job loss. In L. Ferman & J. Gordus (Eds.), *Mental health and the economy.* Kalamazoo, MI: W.E. Upjohn Institute for Employment Research.

Kaufman, H.G. (1982). *Professionals in search of work: Coping with the stress of job loss and underemployment.* NY: John Wiley & Sons.

King, C. (1982, January). *Social impacts of mass layoff* (CRSO Working Paper No. 254). Ann Arbor, MI: University of Michigan, Center for Research on Social Organization.

Kornhauser, A.W. (1965). *Mental health of the industrial worker.* NY: Wiley.

LaRocco, J.M., House, J. & French, J.R.P. (1980). Social support, occupational stress and health. *Journal of Health and Social Behavior, 21,* 202-218.

Liem, R. & Rayman, P. (1982). Health and the social costs of umemployment. *American Psychologist, 37,* 1116-1124.

Parnes, H.S. & King, R. (1977). Middle aged job losers. *Industrial Gerontology, 4,* 77-95.

Powell, D.H., & Driscoll, P.J. (1973). Middle class professionals face unemployment. *Society, 10,* 18-26.

Price, R.H. (1982a February). *Four domains of prevention research.* Paper presented to the National Institute of Mental Health Conference on Prevention, Austin, Texas.

Price, R.H. (1982b). *Priorities for prevention research: Linking risk factor and intervention research.* Washington, D.C.: National Institute of Mental Health, Center for Studies of Prevention.

Price, R.H. (1984). *Research on mental health problems in the worksite: A state of the art review.* Paper presented at the First Business and Industry Roundtable on Alcohol, Drug Abuse and Mental Disorders at the Worksite, Washington, D.C.

Price, R.H. (in press). Work and community. *American Journal of Community Psychology.*

Price, R.H., & Bronfman, L. (1984, September). *Bibliography: Unemployment and occupa-*

tional stress: Risk factors and intervention programs. (Available from The Institute for Social Research, P.O. Box 1248, Ann Arbor, MI 48106-1248).

Price, R.H., Ketterer, R.F., Bader, B.C., & Monahan, J. (Eds.). (1980). *Prevention in community mental health: Research, policy and practice.* Beverly Hills, CA: Sage Publications.

Pursell, D.E. (1980). The beginning of a new era: The transition from a labor surplus to a labor short economy. *Thrust, 2*(2), 243-257.

Schlozman, K.L., & Verba, S. (1979). *Injury to insult: Unemployment, class and political response.* Cambridge, MA: Harvard University Press.

Slote, A. (1969). *Termination: The closing at Baker plant.* Indianapolis, IN: Bobbs-Merrill.

Wortman, P.M. (1983). Evaluation research: A methodological perspective. *Annual Review of Psychology, 34,* 223-260.

Yeaton, W.H., & Wortman, P.M. (Eds.). (in press). Evaluation issues in medical data synthesis. In W.H. Yeaton & P.M. Wortman (Eds.), *Data synthesis, Methodological and conceptual issues.* San Francisco, CA: Jossey-Bass.

Zawadzki, B., & Lazarsfeld, P. (1935, May). The psychological consequences of underemployment. *The Journal of Social Psychology, 6,* 224-251.

Publications

THE MICHIGAN PROGRAM

Michigan Department of Mental Health (1982). Guidelines for continuation and transfer of demonstration projects. *Public mental health administrative manual* (Report No. IV-H-007-0001). Lansing, MI: Author.

Michigan Department of Mental Health (1983). Guidelines for community/caregiver services. *Public mental health administrative manual* (Report No. IV-H-006-0001). Lansing, MI: Author.

Michigan Department of Mental Health (1984). Prevention services. *Public mental health administrative manual* (Report No. IV-H-005-0003). Lansing, MI: Author.

Tableman, B. (1975). *Recommendations for the development of a prevention system.* Lansing: Michigan Department of Mental Health.

The initial plan for the Michigan program, covering administrative and programmatic aspects.

Tableman, B. (1980). Prevention activities at the state level. In R.H. Price (Ed.), *Prevention in mental health* (pp. 237-252). Beverly Hills: Sage Publications.

Describes the development and rationale of the Michigan program.

Tableman, B. (1981) (1982) (1983). *Annual report for the prevention program.* Lansing: Michigan Department of Mental Health.

Tableman, B. (in press). The politics of the possible. In M. Kessler & S. Goldston (Eds.), *Proceedings of the Tenth Annual Vermont Conference on Prevention of Psychopathology.* Hanover: University Press of New England.

Describes the ways in which states have implemented prevention programming and strategic considerations.

SPECIFIC PROJECTS

Children of Disordered Adults

Cohen, E. (1981). *Social competence curriculum for children of disordered adults.* Lansing: Michigan Department of Mental Health. $10.

A discussion of the characteristics of children of disordered adults and a scripted curriculum for teaching interpersonal cogntive problem-solving skills, adapted from the work of M. Shure and of E. Gesten and R. Weissberg.

Infant Mental Health

Michigan Department of Mental Health (1983). Guidelines for infant mental health services. *Public mental health administrative manual* (Report No. IV-H-009-0001). Lansing, MI: Author.

Michigan Department of Mental Health (in press). *Infant mental health services: A replication manual.* Lansing, MI: Author.

Shapiro, V., Adelson, E., & Tableman, B. (1980). Beginning at the beginning: The introduction of infant mental health services to community mental health clinics. In S. Fraiberg (Ed.), *Clinical studies in infant mental health* (pp. 270-279). New York: Basic Books.

A description of the initial training in Michigan of community-based infant mental health specialists.

Shapiro, V., Adelson, E., & Tableman, B. (Eds.) (1982). The introduction of infant mental health services in Michigan. *Infant Mental Health Journal, 3,* 69-139.

Includes articles on development of Michigan's infant mental health programming, linkages to medical settings, and services developed by community mental health.

Tableman, B. (1981). *Infant mental health interventions.* Presentation at Institute XVII on Doing Primary Prevention, American Orthopsychiatric Association, New York.

Descriptions of the Kalamazoo Early Intervention Program.

Tableman, B., & Peterson, M.K. (1981). Identification of newborns in "at risk" situations and home visit intervention. *Prevention of psychosocial disorders in infancy: Emerging perspectives for the 80's: Symposium proceedings* (pp. 34-40). Pittsburgh: University of Pittsburgh First Born Project.

Parent Education for Low Income Families

Mischley, M.J., Mischley, L.A., & Ingold, B.M. (1983). *Parent education for low income families with young children: A replication manual.* Lansing: Michigan Department of Mental Health. $10.

Provides five session script and information on installing the program.

Stress Management Training for Low Income Women

Feis, C., Howard, D., Tableman, B., & Marciniak, D. (1984). *Use of stress management training as an alternative treatment.* Lansing: Michigan Department of Mental Health.

Fields, S. (1980). Know thy stress. *Innovations, 7,* 16-19.

Marciniak, D., & Tableman, B. (1981). *Stress management training for women on public assistance: A replication manual.* Lansing: Michigan Department of Mental Health. $10.

Provides ten session script and information on installing the program.

Tableman, B. (1983). *Stress management training for women on public assistance.* Presentation at NIMH workshop on prevention of depression, San Francisco.

Tableman, B., Marciniak, D., Johnson, D., & Rodgers, R. (1982). Stress management training for women on public assistance. *American Journal of Community Psychology, 10,* 355-365.

Descriptions of the Ionia project.

Unemployment

Alexander, E. (1978). *Job club is people helping people: A facilitator's manual.* Ann Arbor: Washtenaw County Mental Health Services Board. (Available from Michigan Document Depository Libraries).

Jarley, P. (Ed.) (1980). *Response to major layoffs and plant closings: A collection of readings for community mental health agencies.* Lansing: Michigan Department of Mental Health.

State-of-the-art articles as of 1980 covering the mental health impact of unemployment and interventions.

Stone, J., & Kieffer, C. (1984). *Pre-layoff intervention: A response to unemployment.* Ann Arbor: University of Michigan Institute of Science and Technology.

Suggestions for community mental health or other agencies concerned about plant closings and layoffs.

GENERAL ARTICLES

Tableman, B. (1981). Overview of programs to prevent mental health problems of children. *Public Health Reports, 96,* 38-44.

Tableman, B. (1982). Preventive intervention for children and adults. In E. Aronowitz (Ed.), *Prevention strategies for mental health* (pp. 57-80). New York: Prodist.

Reviews of various prevention modalities and illustrative projects.

Tableman, B. (1983). *Adults susceptible to stress-related disorders: Research on prevention initiatives.* Presentation at NIMH NASMHPD Workshops for State Mental Health Directors, Atlanta.

Discussion of four evaluated projects taking different approaches to enhancing management of stress.

INSTRUMENTS

Borgess Interactional Assessment (1981). Kalamazoo: Kalamazoo County Mental Health Services Board.

A checklist to be used by hospital nurses to identify infants in nurturing situations indicative of psycho-social risk. Available from Michigan Department of Mental Health, Prevention and Demonstration Projects.

Objectives/Problems Checklist for Infant Mental Health Services (1984). Lansing: Michigan Department of Mental Health.

Three copy carbon packet, instructions for use, and instructions for simple summary analysis to be used by persons working with infants and families to indicate problems at intake, problems addressed in service plan, and progress made. Available from Michigan Department of Mental Health, Prevention and Demonstration Projects. $10 for initial packet of 30 plus instructions; thereafter, $.25 per unit.

VIDEOTAPES

Chipault, G. (1978). *A better beginning.* Ann Arbor: University of Michigan.

Reviews characteristics of failure-to-thrive infants. Available for rental from Michigan Association for Infant Mental Health, c/o Department of Psychology, Michigan State University, East Lansing, Michigan 48824.

Peterson, M.K. (1978). *Beginnings.* Ann Arbor: University of Michigan.

Presents mother-infant interaction and development of attachment. Available for rental from Michigan Association for Infant Mental Health.

Schelkun, R., Murphy, M., & Cooper, S. (in press). *Managing disruptive individuals in community settings.* Ann Arbor: Washtenaw County Mental Health Services Board.

Three tapes developed with agency input, designed to assist the staff of (1) a library, (2) businesses and organizations serving the public, and (3) other community organizations in managing disruptive individuals. Available for rental from Washtenaw County or from Michigan Department of Mental Health, Prevention and Demonstration Projects.